AEROSOLS AND
THE HUMAN LUNG
An Introduction

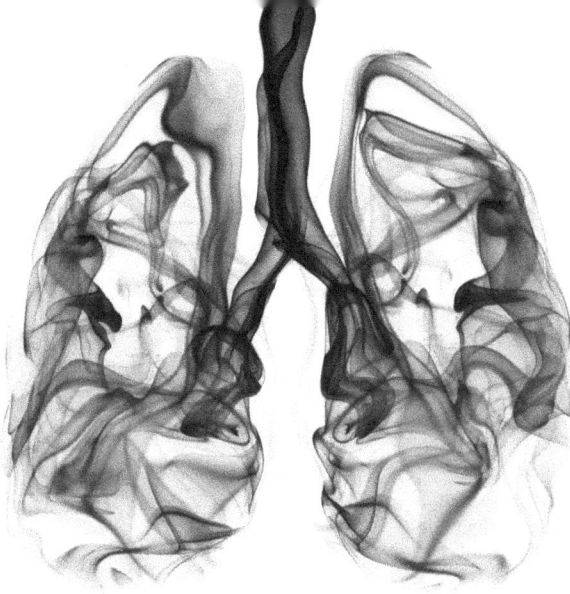

AEROSOLS AND THE HUMAN LUNG
An Introduction

Chantal Darquenne
University of California, San Diego, USA

Otmar Schmid
Helmholtz Zentrum München, Germany

G Kim Prisk
University of California, San Diego, USA

World Scientific

NEW JERSEY · LONDON · SINGAPORE · BEIJING · SHANGHAI · HONG KONG · TAIPEI · CHENNAI · TOKYO

Published by

World Scientific Publishing Co. Pte. Ltd.

5 Toh Tuck Link, Singapore 596224

USA office: 27 Warren Street, Suite 401-402, Hackensack, NJ 07601

UK office: 57 Shelton Street, Covent Garden, London WC2H 9HE

British Library Cataloguing-in-Publication Data

A catalogue record for this book is available from the British Library.

AEROSOLS AND THE HUMAN LUNG
An Introduction

ISBN 978-981-121-217-8 (hardcover)
ISBN 978-981-121-218-5 (ebook for institutions)
ISBN 978-981-121-219-2 (ebook for individuals)

For any available supplementary material, please visit
https://www.worldscientific.com/worldscibooks/10.1142/11604#t=suppl

Typeset by Stallion Press
Email: enquiries@stallionpress.com

Contents

About the Authors   ix

Chapter 1   Introduction   1

   1.1 What Is an Aerosol?   1
   1.2 Aerosols and Breathing   1
   1.3 This Book   4
   References   6

Chapter 2   The Respiratory System   7

   2.1 Structure of the Lung   7
   2.2 Gas Flow in the Airways   11
   2.3 The Pulmonary Circulation and Gas Exchange Barrier   13
   2.4 Airway Wall Structure and Defense   16
   References   18

Chapter 3   Aerosol Transport and Deposition: The Basics   21

   3.1 Characterizing Particle Distributions   21
   3.2 Mechanisms of Aerosol Transport   25
   3.3 Mechanisms of Aerosol Deposition   28
   References   34

Chapter 4   Aerosol Measurement Techniques   **37**

4.1 Introduction   37
4.2 Cascade Impactors   37
4.3 Real-Time Detection and Measurement of Particles   40
4.4 Light Scattering Devices   44
References   48

Chapter 5   Determination of Aerosol Deposition   **49**

5.1 Experimental Determination of Aerosol Deposition   49
5.2 Imaging   59
5.3 Computational Models of Aerosol Deposition   69
References   80

Chapter 6   Clearance of Particles   **87**

6.1 Introduction   87
6.2 Mucociliary Clearance   88
6.3 Macrophages   91
6.4 Translocation to the Interstitium, Lymphatic
      System and/or Blood   92
6.5 Absorption of Soluble Particles   93
6.6 Particle Translocation Beyond the Lungs   93
6.7 Measurement of Particle Clearance   95
References   98

Chapter 7   Aerosols as a Diagnostic Tool   **101**

7.1 Introduction   101
7.2 Aerosol Bolus Dispersion   101
7.3 Aerosol-Based Measurement of Airspace Dimensions   105
References   109

Chapter 8   Aerosol Therapeutics   **113**

8.1 Drugs Classes   113
8.2 Aerosol Delivery Systems   118
References   130

Chapter 9   Ambient and Indoor Aerosol   **133**

9.1 Introduction   133
9.2 Ambient Aerosol   133
9.3 Urban Aerosol   140
9.4 Global Aerosol Emissions   142
9.5 Indoor Aerosol   145
References   148

Chapter 10   Adverse Health Effects of Aerosols   **151**

10.1 Introduction   151
10.2 Linking Aerosol Concentration to Lung-Deposited
      Dose   153
10.3 Evidence for PM-Induced Health Effects   157
10.4 Conclusion   173
References   174

Chapter 11   Aerosols in Unusual Environments   **177**

11.1 Altered Gravity   177
11.2 Aerosols and Planetary Exploration   185
References   190

Chapter 12   Regulation of Particle Exposure   **193**

12.1 Introduction   193
12.2 Guidelines and Regulatory Limits of Particle Exposure   194
12.3 Shifting from Mass- to Surface Area-Derived OELs   199
12.4 Successful PM Mitigation Strategies   204
References   205

Index   207

About the Authors

Chantal Darquenne is a Professor of Medicine at the University of California, San Diego (UCSD). She earned her PhD degree in Applied Sciences from the Université Libre de Bruxelles (Belgium). She completed a postdoctoral fellowship in the Division of Physiology at UCSD where she still holds her current position. Dr Darquenne studies the deposition and dispersion of inhaled aerosols to gain greater insight into the mechanisms involved in particle transport in the lung. Her major research contributions in the field include the study of aerosol inhalation in humans in altered gravity, the development of numerical models that simulate the transport and deposition of aerosols in the lung, the use of Magnetic Resonance Imaging to measure aerosol deposition in animal models, the effect of lung disease such as COPD on both regional and overall aerosol deposition, and the study of upper airway dynamics during breathing and its effect on aerosol transport. She is the President of the International Society for Aerosols in Medicine (2019–2021).

Otmar Schmid is head of the Pulmonary Aerosol Delivery Group at the Helmholtz Zentrum München and the Comprehensive Pneumology Center in Munich, Germany. He is also Adjunct Assistant Professor at the Missouri University of Science and Technology (MST), from which he holds a PhD degree in physics. He has more than 20 years of experience in aerosol science working in the fields of ambient aerosol characterization, combustion aerosols and particle lung deposition. More recently, his research focus has shifted to therapeutic aerosols, dosimetry and biokinetics of aerosols in the lungs and the biological effects of nanoparticles. He holds patents related to aerosol technology and he has worked intensely towards bridging the gap between aerosol science, medicine and toxicology. He has served on the boards of related professional societies including the Association for Aerosol Research (GAeF) and the International Society of Aerosols in Medicine (ISAM).

G Kim Prisk earned his PhD from the University of Otago in 1983 and has been at the University of California, San Diego ever since. He worked extensively on studies of the human lung in weightlessness in spaceflight on both the Space Shuttle and on the International Space Station. These studies were extended to studies on aerosol transport and deposition and the influence of gravity on these processes using parabolic flight. More recently he has worked on the development and use of functional imaging techniques using MRI to quantitatively measure both ventilation and perfusion in the human lung. Despite the low signal to noise environment for MRI in the lung, the techniques offer imaging without the constraints of radiation dose or the use of injected contrast agents, making them well-suited for studies that require repeated imaging. He is an associate editor for the *Journal of Applied Physiology* with an emphasis on pulmonary gas exchange and environmental physiology.

Chapter 1
Introduction

1.1 What Is an Aerosol?

An aerosol is defined as a suspension of solid or liquid particles dispersed in a gas. It is thought that the term *aerosol* was first used during World War 1 to describe an "aero-solution," clouds of microscopic particles in air. While the description above sounds simple enough, there are many details about aerosols that serve to make their properties very different from one case to another. Obviously, the nature of the particles themselves (such as size, mass, and composition) matters, as does the carrying gas. Since aerosols interact with the space in which they are contained (in this case, the lung), their behavior is governed by that space as well. As will become apparent as this book is read, these factors (and others) serve to make the behavior of different aerosols quite distinct from each other.

1.2 Aerosols and Breathing

The focus of this book is the inhalation of aerosols into the human lung. These aerosols can be thought of in two contexts: things we want to be inhaled where a typical example might be an inhaled drug, and things we would rather were not inhaled where an example might be airborne pollutants. Clearly both of these classes of aerosols share a considerable degree of commonality in terms of behavior.

Understanding, studying, and measuring the behavior of an inhaled aerosol requires the combination of aspects of the physical

1

sciences, and of the biological sciences. In terms of the physical sciences, a complete understanding of an inhaled aerosol depends on describing the flow features of the carrier gas, on understanding particle motions such as sedimentation and diffusion, and on the nature and characteristics of the particles such as their size, shape, and hygroscopic properties to name a few. This has to be coupled with an understanding of the human airway tree and how gas flow is distributed within it, a description of the airway lining, and some understanding of the interaction of the particles with the human body once they encounter an airway wall.

The particles that serve to make up an aerosol capable of being inhaled cover a very wide range of sizes from the very large (more than 10 μm in size) to the very small (down to ~0.001 μm or 1 nm, the so-called nanoparticles) (Figure 1.1). Clearly, given this size range

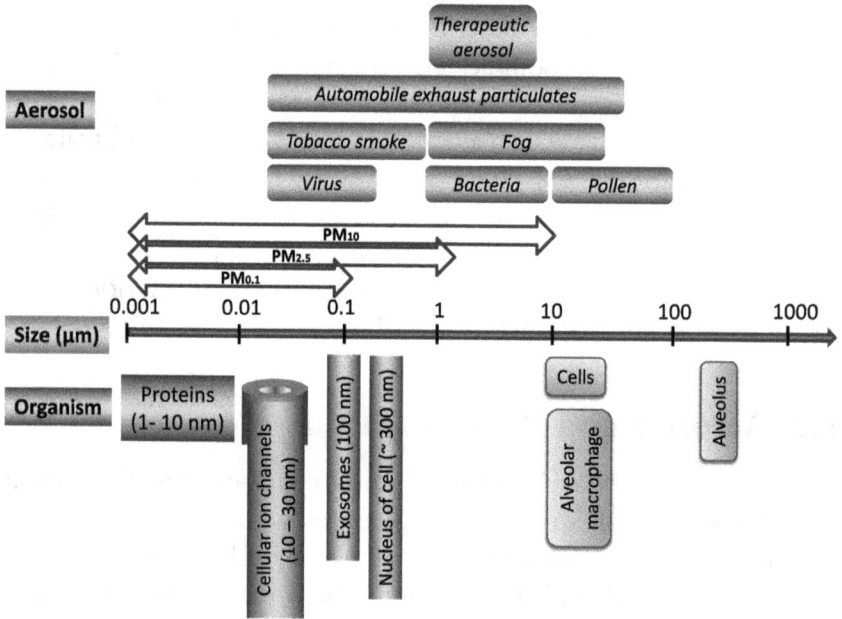

Figure 1.1:   A schematic showing the wide range of sizes of inhaled aerosol particles (~30 μm down to the nanometer scale) with a comparison of the size of key elements that might be found in the human body.

covering more than 4 orders of magnitude, there is no "one-size fits all" approach to understanding the behavior of an inhaled aerosol.

1.2.1 *Aerosolized Drug Delivery*

It is fair to say that the understanding of aerosol behavior in the human lung was greatly advanced by the development and refinement of inhaled drug delivery. Inhalation therapy, typically for diseases such as asthma, has been used for thousands of years, often in the form of herbal smoke inhalation or of some hot medicated vapor inhalation. In the 1800s and early 1900s, "asthma cigarettes" were in widespread use, which was clearly a form of aerosolized drug delivery. Similarly, there were numerous examples of devices designed to administer either liquid aerosols or dry powders for therapeutic purposes.[1]

However, the development and release (in 1956) by Riker Laboratories (now 3M Drug Delivery Systems) of the first pressurized metered dose inhaler (pMDI) for the delivery of isoproterenol and epinephrine began what might be thought of as the modern phase of aerosolized drug delivery. Variants on this theme both in the form of pMDIs and dry powder inhalers are now a universal aspect of asthma therapy and are increasingly used in therapies for other lung diseases and some systemic diseases. As the understanding of aerosol behavior has improved, so too has the innovative nature of these drug delivery devices, with an aim to improve the efficacy of the therapeutic action of the drug, while minimizing side effects.

1.2.2 *Environmental Aerosols*

The other parallel development in the understanding of inhaled aerosols comes from the recognition of the risks associated with environmental aerosols and the concomitant rise in the regulation of these aerosols.

Environmental aerosols result from both natural sources (e.g., forest fires and dust storms) and man-made sources (e.g., industrial activity and automobile exhaust). Industrial activity can provide circumstances when high levels of exposure to aerosols occur (e.g., mining and sandblasting). Air pollution events are often associated with combustion emissions. One of the most famous examples is the great fog of London in 1952, a city-wide pollution event in which atmospheric conditions combined with the use of coal fires for home heating blanketed the city in a thick smog (a combination of smoke and fog) for 6 days. It is thought that this event resulted in more than 4000 excess deaths,[2] and this event was a major driver in the subsequent passing of the Clean Air Act in the United Kingdom in 1956.

As time has passed and our knowledge of the health effects of aerosols has increased, there has been a recognition by regulatory agencies of the need to introduce more stringent standards. This has resulted in reduction in allowable particulate counts, but importantly, more stringent regulation of aerosol particles in smaller size ranges. Early regulations pertaining to total suspended particle loads have transitioned to regulation of PM_{10} (particulate matter less than 10 μm in size) to $PM_{2.5}$ (particulate matter less than 2.5 μm in size) with more recent regulation of $PM_{0.1}$ (particulate matter less than 0.1 μm in size). These standards result from a better understanding of the role played by small particles, an understanding which in turn is a result of better understanding of the transport processes involved.

1.3 This Book

This book is aimed at readers, likely at the graduate student level, entering the field. Such persons will likely come from varied backgrounds, some from the physical sciences and some from the biological sciences. We have tried to provide entry-level information for both.

We have structured this book along the lines laid out in this introductory chapter. We start with a description of the human airway tree (Chapter 2), as this structure serves to greatly influence how particles enter the lung, how they deposit in the lung, how they are cleared from the lung, and how they interact with the lung (and thus the rest of the body itself). This is followed by the basics of aerosol transport and deposition (Chapter 3). This is an aspect of aerosol science where physical sciences dominate and where a basic understanding of fluid dynamics is a useful tool. Because aerosol particles are contained in the gas (typically air), how that air moves directly affects particle transport. There are sophisticated tools for such studies such as computational fluid dynamics, but a basic understanding can be made without resorting to such approaches.

We then turn to means of measuring particle properties themselves (Chapter 4). Since particle size and mass inextricably determine how they interact with the carrier gas flow, it is critical that such measurements can be made. These physical measurements lead to the measurement of aerosol deposition in the human lung (Chapter 5). This brings together the preceding chapters because such deposition depends on particle characteristics, the nature of the airways and gas flow, and if deposition is to be measured, measuring the particles. This necessarily brings into play some imaging techniques, and these are briefly described. The other tool that comes into play in this context is computational models. These have been an essential tool and with time and increased computational power have become ever more comprehensive. Much development and understanding of aerosol deposition has resulted from *in silico* studies. Once deposited, there are clearance mechanisms in the lung (Chapter 6) that serve to remove deposited particles, and these play a critical role in avoiding some of the deleterious effects of the deposited particles.

The next two chapters deal with the use of inert aerosol particles as diagnostic tools (Chapter 7) and the ever-widening role of aerosols as therapeutic agents (Chapter 8). Both these topics depend on aerosol deposition, and the development of improved diagnostic techniques has helped to drive the development of improved drug delivery systems to improve efficacy and minimize side effects.

The last group of chapters deals with the adverse aspects of environmental aerosols. Sources of such aerosols, both natural and man-made, as well as exposure situations, are discussed (Chapter 9). The adverse health effects of environmental aerosols (Chapter 10) are widespread and are both acute and long-term in nature. Such effects drive the regulatory environment as they have the potential to have significant public health consequences. Chapter 11 deals with aerosols in the unusual environment of altered gravity, which although unlikely to be encountered by most people, has contributed considerably to the understanding of how aerosols deposit in the lung and is a potential risk to those undertaking planetary exploration in the future. We finish with a deliberately brief chapter on the governmental and regulatory issues (Chapter 12). As pointed out above, these have evolved considerably over time and will continue to do so in the future. Rather than provide a detailed description of the current regulations, which will inevitably soon become out of date, we have provided key links to the major regulatory agencies in the hope that this will provide a useful portal in the future.

Each chapter is individually referenced so that chapters of interest can be read alone, or in groups as needed.

References

1. Stein SW, and Thiel CG. (2017). The history of therapeutic aerosols: A chronological review. *J. Aerosol Med. Pulm. Drug Deliv.* **30**: 20–41.
2. Wilson R, and Spengler J. (1996). Introduction. In: *Particles in our Air: Concentrations and Health Effects.* Harvard School of Public Health, pp. 1–14.

Chapter 2
The Respiratory System

2.1 Structure of the Lung

In much the same way that Christmas ornaments are best appreciated when hung on a Christmas tree, a discussion of the critical elements of aerosol transport in the lung (the ornaments) is perhaps best approached by having a framework on which to hang them (the tree). In that spirit, we will outline the structure of the lung and the consequences of that structure in relation to aerosol transport.

The structure of the human lung stems directly from the constraints imposed by the volume of space available for the lung to occupy, gas transport, and the gas exchange mechanism itself. Of these elements, the principal factor that determines the anatomy of the mammalian lung stems from the fact that gas exchange occurs through the process of passive diffusion. Passive diffusion, wherein gas transport occurs down a gradient of partial pressure, requires no external energy source (in contrast to, for example, active ion transport occurring in the kidney), but requires a large surface area and a very thin transport barrier to work efficiently. It is the combination of these requirements (large diffusive surface area and thin diffusive membrane), which must be satisfied simultaneously, that "drives" the anatomy of the lung. This structure in turn serves to greatly influence aerosol transport, aerosol deposition, and the eventual fate of inhaled aerosol particles.

The result of these requirements is a gas exchange organ (the lung) with a gas exchanging surface area of ~50–100 m^2 and a diffusive membrane, the blood–gas barrier, with a thickness of ~ 0.3 μm.[1-3] The huge surface area of the lung (approximately the area of one side of a tennis court) means that lung epithelium presents by far the greatest surface area to the outside environment of any organ, and the structure that leads to this (described in the following section) has important implications in terms of where inhaled aerosol particles deposit in the lung. The incredibly thin alveolar capillary membrane also carries with it important implications in terms of the translocation of deposited particles from the lung to other organs in the body (described in Chapter 6).

2.1.1 *The Extra-thoracic Airways*

To reach the lung, inhaled gas or aerosol must first traverse the extra-thoracic airways, often referred to as the upper airways. Those parts of this anatomy above the beginning of the trachea are shown in Figure 2.1. As gas is inhaled either through the complex pathways of the nose or through the mouth, it is warmed and wetted by the

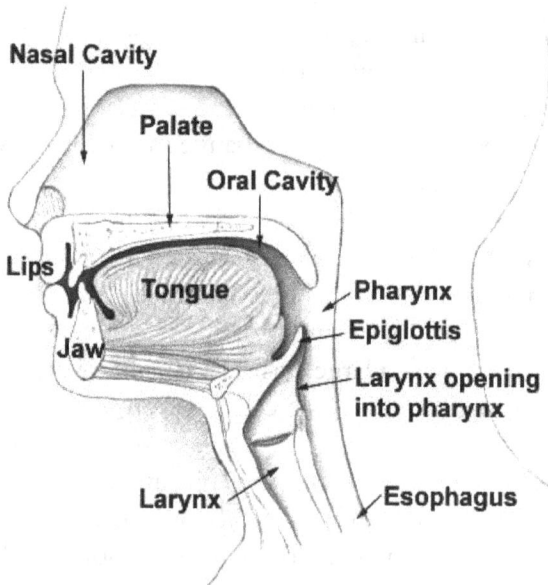

Figure 2.1: The extra-thoracic or upper airways. Inhaled gas and aerosol must traverse this part of the anatomy before reaching the trachea.

Source: https://training.seer.cancer.gov/head-neck/anatomy/overview.html. US Government web site. Images are public domain

presence of the mucus membrane. This is an important point when considering hygroscopic aerosols as this has the capability to result in particle size growth. The gas passes through the pharyngeal regions and then through the larynx that forms the upper boundary of the trachea.

The geometry of the nasal turbinates is complicated, and this region serves to provide an efficient filtering mechanism to reduce the number of aerosol particles that reach the lung. Defining the effect of this geometry on aerosol transport is difficult, but there are several examples of *in vitro* models that have been developed for this purpose.[4-7] In this context, it is also worth noting that the nasal passages of rodents such as mice and rats (which are obligate nose breathers) are much more efficient at filtering inhaled aerosols than the nasal passages of humans. This serves to make inhaled deposition studies in rodents somewhat more difficult.

2.1.2 *The Airway Tree*

The challenge of fitting 50–100 m² of membrane into a thoracic volume (at rest) of approximately 2–3 L is met by dividing that volume into millions of tiny air sacs (alveoli). Original estimates of the number of alveoli in the human were ~300 million,[2] but subsequent work has raised that number to an average of ~480 million.[1] Each alveolus is on average ~200 μm in diameter so that ~170 alveoli can be found in a single cubic millimeter of lung. Overall, this provides a lung with a total surface area of ~60 m², a number that falls within the previous estimate of 50–100 m².

To connect each alveolus to the outside world for gas exchange, a branching network of airways forms the basic structure of the lung (Figure 2.2). In humans, this tree is in the form of a fairly regular branching dichotomy, where each airway splits into two somewhat equal daughter branches, at relatively similar branching angles. In this sense, the airway tree resembles many branching deciduous trees (e.g. an oak tree) where the trunk of the tree is analogous to the trachea. It is also worth noting that the regular dichotomy of the human lung is not the norm in most other mammalian lungs (such as the sheep and pig), which tend to have a more dominant main airway from

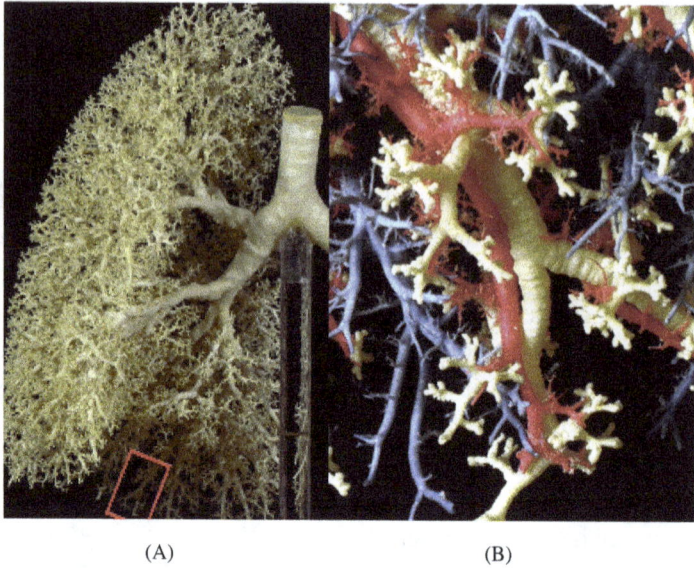

(A)   (B)

Figure 2.2: (A) Silicone rubber casts of the airways of the human lung (in white).[8] (B) Casts in a region approximately the size of the red box in (A) that include airways (white), pulmonary arteries (red), and pulmonary veins (blue). Note the similarity of the branching structures. The pulmonary arteries accompany the airways, while the pulmonary veins are located "between" airway branches. Used with permission from Ref. 8.

which small branches depart, more closely resembling a pine tree. These are often referred to as monopodal branching patterns. This seemingly minor point may carry some importance when considering studies performed in animal lungs with the intention of inferring aerosol behavior in the human lung.

This regular dichotomous branching pattern in humans led to a simplified description of the airway tree by Weibel[3] and subsequently updated in which the trachea was considered as generation zero, and with each succeeding bifurcation, the number of airways doubled (Figure 2.3). In this model, there are 23 generations after the trachea with alveoli appearing in the model at generation 15. This provides a useful splitting of the model into the conducting zone, generations 0–14, which play no part in gas exchange, but rather just serve as conduits to conduct air, and generations 15–23, the respiratory zone, where all gas exchange occurs.

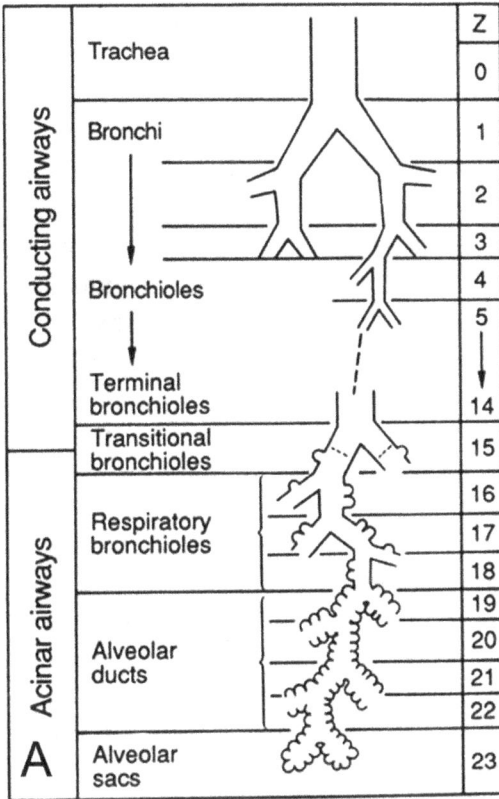

Figure 2.3: A highly simplified but useful model describing the structure of the human airway tree. Each generation divides into two daughter branches that are smaller in size. This regular dichotomy continues for ~23 generations. The zone down to generation 14 contains no gas exchange units (alveoli) and is termed the conducting zone. Alveolarization begins at approximately generation 15. Used with permission from Ref. 8.

Despite the obvious simplifying assumptions built into this model, it remains a useful means to describe the human airway tree.

2.2 Gas Flow in the Airways

The cast of an airway tree shown in Figure 2.2, in which the alveoli are pruned away, is representative of generations 0 to ~16 and thus shows only the conducting part of the lung. This is used to transport gas to the alveoli; no gas exchange occurs in the regions of the lung shown in the cast. Airflow in the lung is reciprocal in nature; gas is both inspired and expired along the same pathway. As a consequence, the last amount of fresh gas taken in during inspiration fills the conducting airways and remains there until expired, never reaching the alveoli where gas exchange occurs. Similarly, the last amount of exhaled gas from the alveoli remains in the conducting airways and is thus re-inspired as the next inspiration begins. The volume of the conducting airways in a normal adult is ~150 mL and is termed the *anatomic* dead space — a part of the lung that receives air but does not participate in gas exchange. However, despite the name — dead space — this region remains very important in the context of aerosol deposition in the lung, and the reciprocal nature of airflow through the conducting airways provides opportunities for particle deposition during BOTH inspiration and expiration.

A very important consequence of this branching structure is that when moving from the trachea to the distal generations of airway branches, there is a huge increase in the total cross-sectional area of the airways. While each daughter airway generation is smaller than the parent, the bifurcating structure means that at each generation, the number of airways doubles (Figure 2.3). The consequence is a rapid increase in the total airway cross-sectional area (Figure 2.4), so that when the end of the airway tree is reached, a huge cross-sectional area is available for gas exchange. This large area is critical for the process of passive diffusion, which is responsible for pulmonary gas exchange.

In terms of the transport of inhaled aerosols, the rapid increase in airway cross-sectional area means that the forward convective velocity of gas during inspiration falls rapidly as the periphery of the lung is approached. As aerosol particles are carried by this convective flow (for the most part, the particles in the micron-size range are so massive that Brownian diffusion is not an effective transport mechanism), and as the end of the airways seen in Figure 2.2 is approached, the forward velocity of the particles in the airflow falls precipitously. For the inspired gas molecules that need to reach the

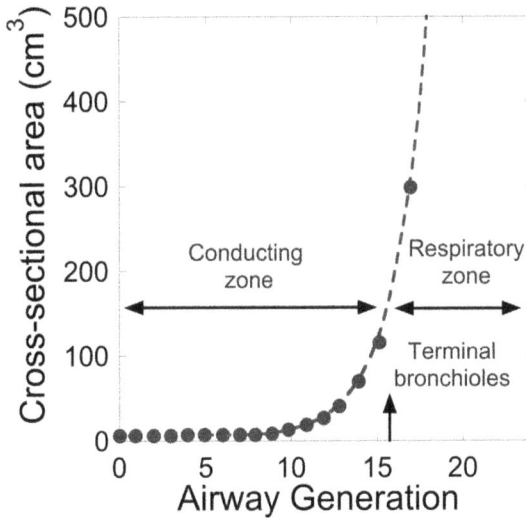

Figure 2.4: Calculated cross-section of the cumulative airway tree from the Weibel A model. Although each daughter branch is smaller than the parent, the number doubles with each successive bifurcation. The consequence is that as the respiratory zone is reached, there is a tremendous increase in the total cross-sectional area, so that by the end of the airway (~generation 23), the total cross-sectional area has expanded from a few cm^2 to 50–100 m^2. Modified from Ref. 9.

alveolar-capillary membrane, gas phase diffusion becomes the dominant form of gas transport from approximately generation 16 onward, but this does not greatly affect inhaled particles. Chapter 3 discusses these processes in detail.

2.3 The Pulmonary Circulation and Gas Exchange Barrier

Both the pulmonary arteries and the pulmonary veins have a bifurcating structure closely mimicking the airways. Along most of their length, the pulmonary arteries accompany the airways, while the pulmonary veins are somewhat offset, lying in the lung parenchyma between pairs of arteries/airways.

The pulmonary arteries and veins are joined to each other through the pulmonary capillaries. As the airways begin to have

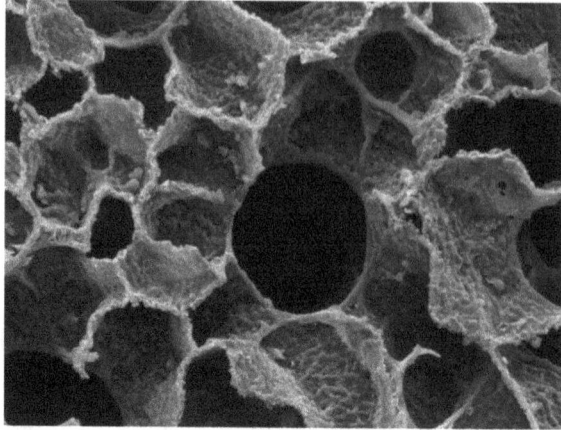

Figure 2.5:   Scanning electron micrograph of the alveoli surrounding an airway.[11] Note that the capillary bed essentially forms the alveolar wall so that the entire surface area of the alveolus participates in gas exchange. Used with permission from Ref. 11.

alveoli in their walls (generation 16 in the Weibel model of airways) (Figure 2.3), their rapid budding forms what is referred to as the pulmonary acinus. This unit of lung is a small independent region of lung ~5 mm across[10,11] with a volume of 150–170 mm^3, and is the region of the lung where gas exchange occurs. All the airways ultimately terminate in alveoli contained within the acinus, and each of these alveoli is in the form of a cavity ~0.2 mm across,[1] the walls of which are entirely covered with pulmonary capillaries (Figure 2.5). Thus, while there are a large number of alveoli in the human lung (~480,000,000), the number of pulmonary capillaries is very much greater, as each alveolus has wall composed almost entirely of pulmonary capillaries (Figure 2.6). The capillaries are ~7–10 μm in diameter, which is just large enough for a red blood cell to squeeze through (see Figure 2.6).

The thin sheet of blood covering each alveolus must be separated from the air space within each alveolus, and this is the job of the alveolar-capillary membrane, often referred to as the blood–gas barrier. This barrier is shown in Figure 2.7. This transmission electron micrograph shows a pulmonary capillary in cross section. The open spaces near the edge of the image are airspaces within an alveolus. The

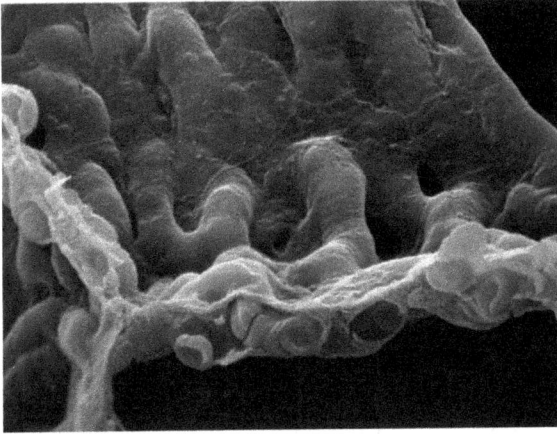

Figure 2.6: High magnification view of the alveolar wall showing the dense capillary network.[11] Red blood cells can be seen within the capillaries. Note that capillaries are sufficiently small so that red blood cells essentially pass through in a serial fashion, forming an effective monolayer, minimizing the distance (and thus the thickness) that O_2 must pass through as it moves from the alveolar space into the red blood cell. Used with permission from Ref. 11.

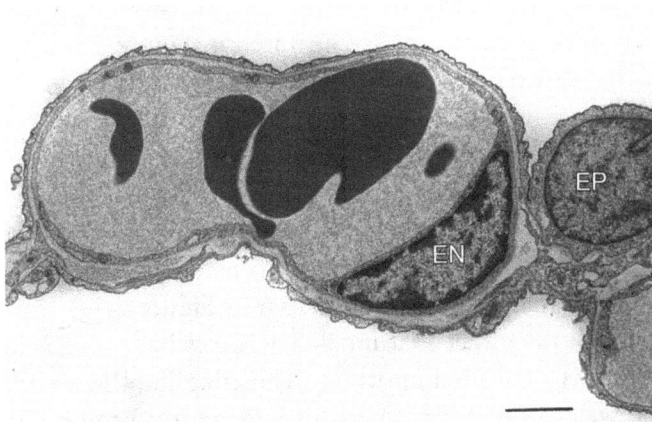

Figure 2.7: Transmission electron micrograph of a single pulmonary capillary in cross section. The white area outside the capillary is the alveolar airspace with the red blood cell inside the capillary caught in cross section. Gas exchange occurs along the arrow moving from the alveolar space, through the epithelial layer (EP), the basement membrane (BM), and the endothelial layer (EM). The nucleus of the endothelial cell (EN) and the epithelial cell (EP) are marked. The scale bar is 1 μm. Used with permission from Ref. 8.

dark object is a red blood cell cut in cross section, and this is contained within a pulmonary capillary. O_2 must cross from the alveolar space to the interior of the red blood cell for transport to the tissues of the body. The alveolar epithelial cell extensions that form the air-exposed walls of the alveolus (labeled EP), the interstitial layer that is composed of the basement membrane of the alveolar wall (the "scaffolding" of the alveolus), and the capillary endothelial cell extensions that form the inside of the capillary wall (EN) separate blood from air. Remarkably, these three barrier layers together comprise a wall thickness of only ~0.3 μm.

The extreme thinness of the blood–gas barrier at times allows very small particles (typically in the nanometer size range) that have deposited in the alveoli to translocate, through the blood–gas barrier to the pulmonary circulation. From there, they can be transported to other locations in the body. This topic is explored more in Chapter 6.

2.4 Airway Wall Structure and Defense

As one traverses the airways from the trachea toward the alveoli, the airway wall structure changes as illustrated in Figure 2.8.

The large central airways are supported by cartilaginous rings to promote lumen stability. There are mucus glands that secrete the mucus layer that lines the airways. Once one progresses beyond approximately generation 6, the airways become thinner-walled, without cartilage. By the time the alveoli are reached, the wall becomes very thin, without cilia, and ultimately becomes the incredibly thin gas exchange membrane shown in Figure 2.7.

In terms of the effect that inhaled aerosols have on the lung, the ciliary system is critically important. The cilia line the airways virtually all the way to the point where alveolarization begins. These cilia beat in a coordinated fashion within a 2-layer mucus system where the lower level (nearer the epithelium) is a lower viscosity layer (the sol layer), over which is a more viscous gel layer (Figure 2.9). The cilia in the airways beat so that the transport direction is towards the epiglottis. In the upper airways (e.g., in the nose), they beat such

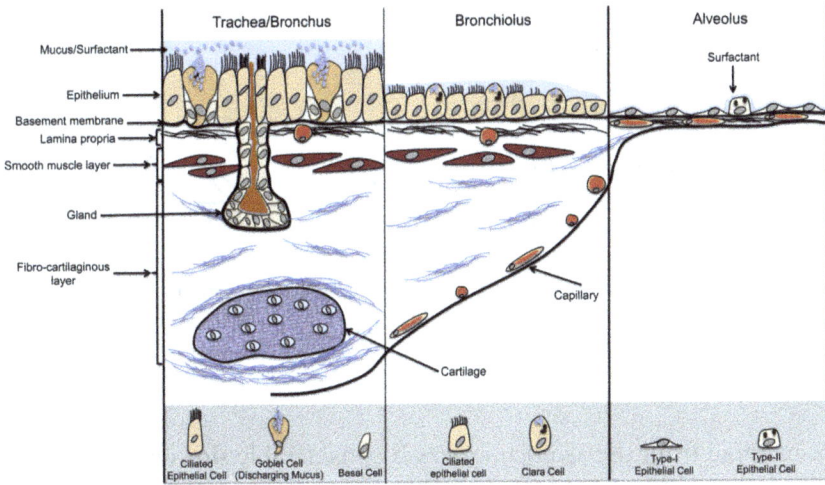

Figure 2.8: The changing structure of the airway wall with location. In the large airways (labeled Trachea/Bronchus), the airway is supported by cartilaginous rings and lined with columnar epithelial cells. Mucus glands secrete a mucus layer that sits on top of a layer of cilia. In the small airways towards the periphery (labeled Bronchiolus), the cartilage is absent, the epithelial cells are more cuboid, and the airway wall becomes much thinner, bringing the capillaries into closer proximity to the airway. Once the alveolus is reached, the wall consists of essentially nothing more than a sandwich of type I epithelial cells, a basement membrane layer, and capillary endothelium as shown in Figure 2.6. There are no cilia in this region. In the alveolar region, there are also type II alveolar epithelial cells that produce pulmonary surfactant, a substance that lowers surface tension, promoting alveolar stability. Occasional goblet cells that secrete mucus are not shown. Used with permission from Ref. 12.

that transport is again towards the epiglottis with the result that foreign particles deposited in any location move towards the epiglottis where the mucus and the deposited particles are swallowed and eliminated.

Particles that deposit in the alveolar region, beyond the extent of the mucociliary clearance system, are cleared from the lung much more slowly through phagocytosis by alveolar macrophages. These cells slowly move around the alveoli engulfing foreign material for subsequent disposal. As a direct consequence, the rapidity of removal

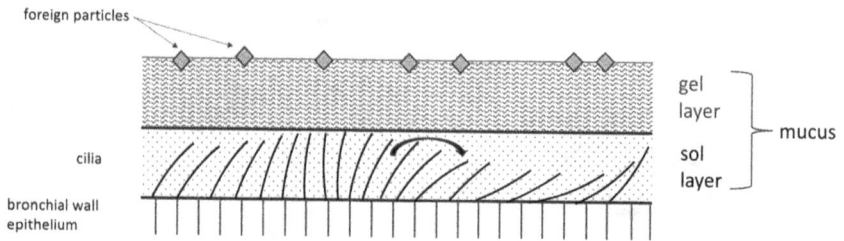

Figure 2.9:   Illustration of the structure of the mucociliary system. The mucus layer is composed of 2 sub-layers, the lower (sol layer) having lower viscosity. The cilia beat within this layer, moving the sticky gel layer forward.

of material from the alveolar spaces is considerably slower than that of material deposited in the ciliated airways. Chapter 6 discusses these processes in detail.

References

1. Ochs M, Nyengaard JR, Jung A, Knudsen L, Voigt M, Wahlers T, Richter J, and Gundersen HJ. (2004). The number of alveoli in the human lung. *Am. J. Respir. Crit. Care Med.* **169**: 120–124.
2. Weibel ER, and Gomez DM. (1962). Architecture of the human lung. Use of quantitative methods establishes fundamental relations between size and number of lung structures. *Science* **137**: 577–585.
3. Weibel ER, (1963). *Morphometry of the Human Lung.* New York: Academic Press.
4. Grgic B, Finlay WH, Burnell PKP, and Heenan AF. (2004). *In vitro* intersubject and intrasubject deposition measurements in realistic mouth-throat geometries. *J. Aerosol Sci.* **35**: 1025–1040.
5. Byron PR, Hindle M, Lange CF, Longest PW, McRobbie D, Oldham MJ, Olsson B, Thiel CG, Wachtel H, and Finlay WH. (2010). *In vivo–in vitro* correlations: Predicting pulmonary drug deposition from pharmaceutical aerosols. *J. Aerosol Med. Pulm. Drug Deliv.* **23 Suppl 2**: S59–S69.
6. Golshahi L, Vehring R, Noga ML, and Finlay WH. (2013). *In vitro* deposition of micrometer-sized particles in the extrathoracic airways of children during tidal oral breathing. *J. Aerosol Sci.* **57**: 14–21.

7. Chen JZ, Katz IM, Pichelin M, Zhu K, Caillibotte G, Noga ML, Finlay WH, and Martin AR. (2017). Comparison of pulsed versus continuous oxygen delivery using realistic adult nasal airway replicas. *Int. J. Chron. Obstruct. Pulmon. Dis.* **12**: 2559–2571.

8. Weibel ER. (2013). It takes more than cells to make a good lung. *Am. J. Respir. Crit. Care Med.* **187**: 342–346.

9. West JB. (2012). *Respiratory Physiology — The Essentials.* Baltimore: Lippincott Williams & Wilkins.

10. Sapoval B, Filoche M, and Weibel ER. (2002). Smaller is better — but not too small: A physical scale for the design of the mammalian pulmonary acinus. *Proc. Natl. Acad. Sci. U. S. A.* **99**: 10411–10416.

11. Weibel ER, Sapoval B, and Filoche M. (2005). Design of peripheral airways for efficient gas exchange. *Respir. Physiol. Neurobiol.* **148**: 3–21.

12. Klein SG, Hennen J, Serchi T, Blomeke B, and Gutleb AC. (2011). Potential of coculture *in vitro* models to study inflammatory and sensitizing effects of particles on the lung. *Toxicol. In Vitro* **25**: 1516–1534.

Chapter 3
Aerosol Transport and Deposition: The Basics

3.1 Characterizing Particle Distributions

The extent, distribution and site of aerosol deposition are major determinants in the therapeutic or health effects of inhaled aerosols. Aerosols are usually polydisperse, i.e., they contain a wide range of particle sizes. While environmental aerosols present a multimodal size distribution, aerosolized drugs can often be characterized by a single lognormal distribution. Size being one of the most important particle characteristics affecting the fate of inhaled aerosols, it is essential to be able to characterize the size distribution of common aerosols.

Particles can be characterized either by their geometric diameter (d_g) or aerodynamic diameter (d_{ae}). The aerodynamic diameter of an irregular particle is defined as the diameter of a spherical particle with a density of 1 g/cm^3 that has the same settling velocity as the irregular particle. The aerodynamic diameter is also useful for nonunit density spherical particles. For example, a 2 μm-diameter spherical particle with a density of 3 g/cm^3 has similar aerodynamic properties as a unit-density particle with a geometric diameter of 3.5 μm.

When all particles have the same size, the aerosol is called monodisperse. However, most environmental and medical aerosols are polydisperse and are described in terms of a frequency distribution of particle number, mass or surface area as a function of particle diameter (d_p), with d_p being either the geometric or aerodynamic diameter. The

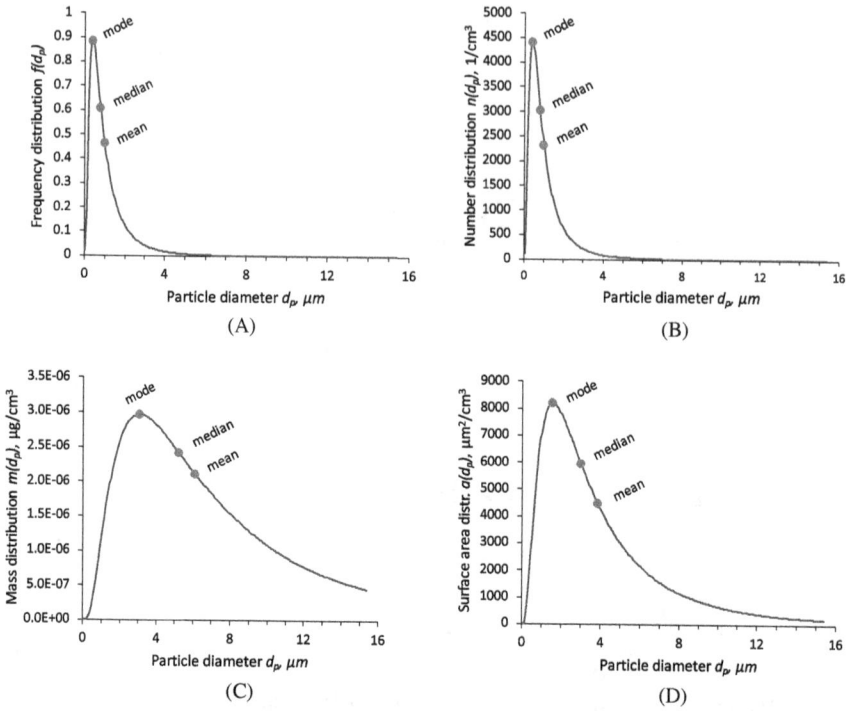

Figure 3.1: Lognormal particle size distributions based on the same frequency distribution and a particle concentration of 5000/cm³. (A) Frequency distribution. (B) Number distribution. (C) Mass distribution. (D) Surface area distribution.

count or number distribution $n(d_p)$ with typical units of $1/\text{cm}^3$ is defined as

$$n(d_p) = N \cdot f(d_p) \tag{3.1}$$

where N is the total number of particles and $f(d_p)$ is the frequency distribution curve (Figure 3.1A):

$$df = f(d_p) \cdot dd_p \tag{3.2}$$

with df representing the fraction of particles with a diameter between d_p and $d_p + dd_p$. An example of number distribution $n(d_p)$ is shown in Figure 3.1B.

Because the mass of the particles has a significant effect on their dynamic properties, it is often more useful to describe inhaled aerosols in terms of their mass distribution (Figure 3.1C). Assuming spherical particles, the mass concentration for particles with a diameter between d_p and $d_p + \mathrm{d}d_p$ is

$$\mathrm{d}m = m(d_p) \cdot \mathrm{d}d_p \qquad (3.3)$$

$$\mathrm{d}m = \frac{\pi}{6} \cdot \rho_p \cdot n(d_p) \cdot d_p^3 \cdot \mathrm{d}d_p \qquad (3.4)$$

where $m(d_p)$ is the mass of a particle with diameter d_p and ρ_p is the particle density. Thus, the mass distribution is

$$m(d_p) = \frac{\pi}{6} \cdot \rho_p \cdot d_p^3 \cdot n(d_p) \qquad (3.5)$$

A third distribution commonly used is the surface area distribution $a(d_p)$ as it has been proposed that surface area is a more appropriate indicator than mass for evaluating efficacy of inhaled drugs or for evaluating pulmonary inflammatory responses from exposure to toxic and/or environmental aerosols (Figure 3.1D). The surface area distribution is expressed as

$$a(d_p) = \pi \cdot d_p^2 \cdot n(d_p) \qquad (3.6)$$

Three parameters are commonly used to characterize size distributions: the mean, the median and the mode (Figure 3.1). The mean is calculated as the arithmetic average diameter of the distribution; the median corresponds to the particle diameter that separates the distribution in half with 50% of the particles having a diameter less than the median and thus 50% of the particles having a diameter larger than the median; the mode is the diameter that corresponds to the maximum frequency in the distribution. The values of these parameters differ between the number, mass and surface area distributions so it is important to know which distribution they are derived from (Table 3.1). Also, for the mass distribution, the median is usually referred to as the mass median diameter (MMD) if the distribution is based on the geometric diameter or mass median aerodynamic

Table 3.1: Comparison of arithmetic mean, median and mode for the number, mass and surface area distributions shown in Figure 3.1.

Particle diameter	Mean (μm)	Median (μm)	Mode (μm)
Number distribution	1	0.77	0.38
Mass distribution	6.10	5.24	3.09
Surface area distribution	3.86	2.99	1.54

diameter (MMAD) if the distribution is based on the aerodynamic diameter. The MMAD of an inhaled aerosol is one of the most commonly used diameters.

Finally, the spread of the distribution is assessed by the standard deviation:

$$\sigma = \frac{1}{N}\sqrt{\int_0^\infty (d_p - \text{mean})^2\, n(d_p)\, dd_p} \tag{3.7}$$

where N is the total number of particles and $n(d_p)$ is the number distribution. Similar relationships can be used for the surface area and mass distributions. Another useful parameter is the geometric standard deviation (GSD), which can be shown to be equal to the exponential of σ.

3.1.1 Lognormal Distribution

As mentioned above, aerosols can often be approximated by a lognormal distribution. The lognormal mass distribution is expressed as

$$m(d_{ae}) = \frac{1}{d_{ae}\sqrt{2\pi}}\, exp\left[\frac{-(\ln d_{ae} - \ln \text{MMAD})^2}{2(\ln \text{GSD})^2}\right] \tag{3.8}$$

For a lognormal distribution, 68% of the aerosol mass is contained between the values of MMAD × GSD and MMAD/GSD. It can be shown that these limits correspond on a plot of cumulative mass distribution to the diameters d_{16} and d_{84} below which 16% and 84% of total mass are contained, respectively (Figure 3.2). Thus, GSD can be expressed as

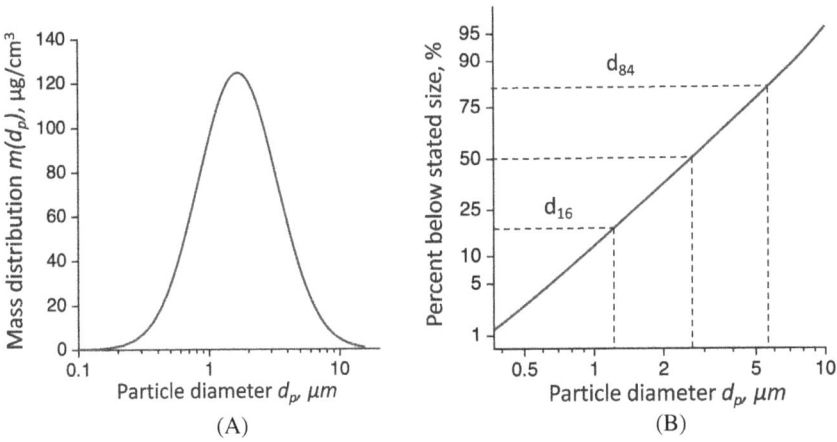

Figure 3.2: Lognormal mass distribution (panel A) and cumulative plot showing the parameters used to define the geometrical standard deviation GSD (panel B). Mode = 1.7 μm; mean = 2.6 μm; median = 2.7 μm; GSD = 2.0, σ = 0.7 μm.

$$\text{GSD} = \sqrt{\frac{d_{84}}{d_{16}}} \qquad (3.9)$$

An aerosol containing particles of the same size has a GSD of 1. In practice, an aerosol with a GSD < 1.22 is considered to be mono-disperse and an aerosol with a GSD ≥ 1.22 is polydisperse.

3.2 Mechanisms of Aerosol Transport

Particle transport in the lung is mainly governed by the gas flow patterns and the particle physical characteristics (size, shape, density). Gas flow patterns and regimes vary widely from the proximal airways to the lung periphery. As mentioned in Chapter 2, while the airways become gradually shorter and narrower with each generation (Figure 2.2), the increasing number of airways with increasing generation number leads to a large increase in the total airway cross-section towards the lung periphery (Figure 2.4). An important consequence in terms of aerosol transport is that this cross-sectional increase results in a large decrease in airflow velocity from the first airway generations down to the periphery of the lung. Accordingly,

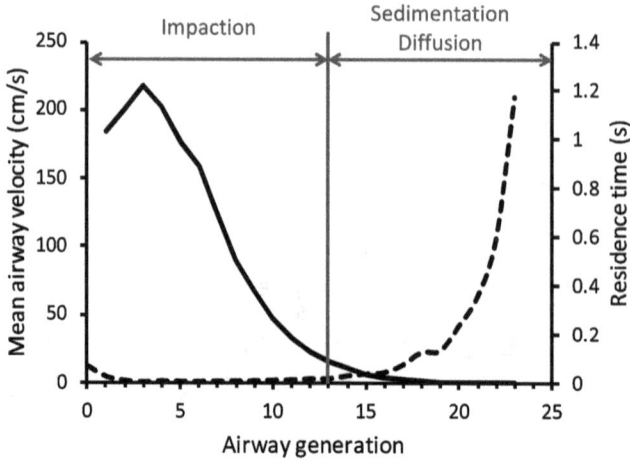

Figure 3.3: Mean airway velocity (solid line) and residence time (dashed line) in the airways as a function of generations of an idealized dichotomous branching lung model (Figure 2.3). As a result, the most relevant mechanism for aerosol deposition onto the lung epithelium changes from impaction in the upper airway generations to sedimentation and diffusion in the lower airway generations (see text for details). Data were calculated for an inspiratory flow rate of 450 mL/s. (Modified from Ref. 1.)

even with the decrease in airway length from proximal to peripheral airways, the residence time in each generation increases with each generation (Figure 3.3). The change in mean airway velocity from the upper airway down to the lung periphery is also accompanied by a change in flow regime.

Flow regime is characterized by the Reynolds number *Re*, a dimensionless parameter describing the relative importance of inertial to viscous forces, expressed as

$$Re = \frac{\rho u d}{\mu} \tag{3.10}$$

where ρ and μ are the gas density and gas dynamic viscosity, respectively, u is the mean flow velocity in the airway and d is the airway diameter. In a cylindrical airway, flow is laminar for $Re < 2100$.[2] When Re increases above 2100, transition to turbulence will occur. During quiet and moderate breathing (flow < 500 mL/s), Reynolds number throughout the intrathoracic airways is below 2100, suggesting laminar flow within the lung. Yet, before reaching the trachea, the inhaled gas is transported through the upper airway that is characterized by drastic changes in cross-sectional areas with a major constriction located at the level of the glottis. Such constriction generates the laryngeal jet, which produces local turbulences that are propagated further down the bronchial tree over several generations of airways, even for local Reynolds number below 2100, before being completely dissipated.[3,4] Indeed, the airway length over these generations is too short to allow the flow to reestablish a laminar profile before the next bifurcation arise, i.e., the length of the airway l is shorter than the so-called entrance length l_E, a measure of the distance required by the flow to be fully developed. The entrance length is a function of airway diameter d and Reynolds number Re.[2] A schematic of the lung along with the flow regime and the ratio of airway to entrance length is shown in Figure 3.4 where parabolic conditions occur once $l/l_E > 1$.

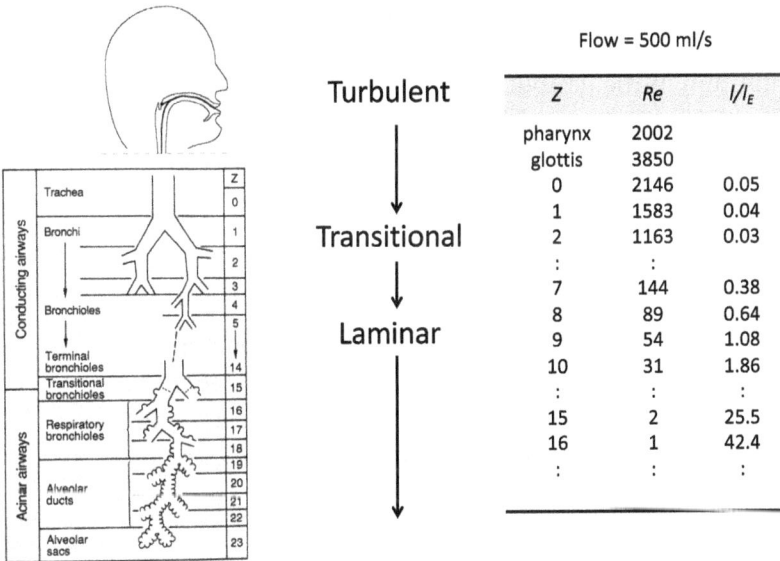

		Flow = 500 ml/s		
	Turbulent	z	Re	l/l_E
		pharynx	2002	
		glottis	3850	
		0	2146	0.05
		1	1583	0.04
	Transitional	2	1163	0.03
		:	:	
		7	144	0.38
		8	89	0.64
	Laminar	9	54	1.08
		10	31	1.86
		:	:	:
		15	2	25.5
		16	1	42.4
		:	:	:

Figure 3.4:   Flow regimes in the human lung during quiet breathing (500 mL/s). The table lists Reynolds number and the ratio of airway length to entrance length as a function of generation number Z. Laminar conditions occur once the airway length becomes longer than the entrance length ($l/l_E > 1$). See text for details.

In addition to gas flow characteristics, aerosol transport is signifi-cantly affected by the intrinsic properties of the particles. Such transport can be described by the Langevin equation, a representation of the 2nd law of Newton that states that the product of the mass of the particle and its acceleration equals the sum of all external forces acting on the particle. These external forces are the drag force ($\vec{F}_D$), the gravitational force ($\vec{F}_G$) and a random force ($\vec{F}_R$) representative of the Brownian motions of the particle. The particle trajectory is thus described by

$$m_p \frac{d\vec{u}_p}{dt} = \vec{F}_D + \vec{F}_G + \vec{F}_R \qquad (3.11)$$

$$m_p \frac{d\vec{u}_p}{dt} = -\frac{3\pi\mu d_p}{C}\left(\vec{u}_p - \vec{u}_f\right) + m_p\vec{g} + F_R(t) \qquad (3.12)$$

where $\vec{u}_p$ and $\vec{u}_f$ are the particle and surrounding fluid velocities, respectively, g is the gravitational acceleration and C is the Cunningham correction factor that accounts for the decreased air resistance caused by slippage when the particle diameter comes close to the mean free path of the gas molecules so that the particle no longer moves as a continuum in the gas but as a particle among discrete gas molecules.[5] Depending on the particle size, some of the external forces may be neglected. This is discussed in the next section along with the main mechanisms of aerosol deposition.

3.3 Mechanisms of Aerosol Deposition

The main mechanisms affecting aerosol transport and deposition in the human lung include inertial impaction, gravitational sedimenta-tion and Brownian diffusion and to a lesser extent turbulent flow, electrostatic precipitation and in the case of elongated particles, inter-ception (Figure 3.5).

3.3.1 *Main Deposition Mechanisms*

3.3.1.1 *Inertial impaction*

Inertial impaction stems from the inability of particles to follow abrupt changes in gas flow direction because of their momentum.

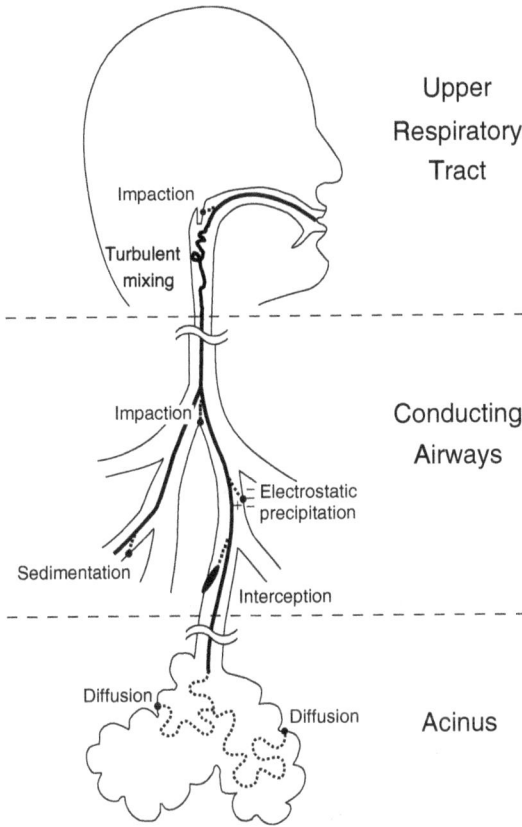

Figure 3.5: Deposition mechanisms of inhaled particles in the lung. Sites of deposition are illustrative but can also occur in other areas of the lung. For example, sedimentation also occurs in the alveolar zone of the lung (see text for details). From Darquenne[6] (Reproduced with permission from the International Society for Aerosols in Medicine (ISAM)).

The probability that a particle will diverge from the air streamlines can be expressed as a function of the Stokes number (*Stk*) defined by

$$Stk = \frac{\rho_p d_p^2 u}{18\mu d} \qquad (3.13)$$

The higher the Stokes' number, the more efficient is the inertial transport and the more likely a particle will deposit by inertial impaction. This velocity-dependent mechanism occurs preferentially in the first few generations of airways where gas and particle velocities are high (Figure 3.3). Inertial impaction is the primary deposition mechanism for particles larger than 5 μm.

3.3.1.2 *Gravitational sedimentation*

Gravitational sedimentation denotes the settling of the particles under the action of gravity g (= 9.81 m/s²; gravitational acceleration). The terminal settling of a particle (V_s) is

$$V_s = \frac{\rho_p d_p^2 u}{18\mu} g \qquad (3.14)$$

Deposition by gravitational sedimentation is proportional to the settling velocity and increases with increasing particle size. As it is a time-dependent mechanism, it is most efficient in the lung periphery where airspace size is small and residence time is high (Figure 3.3). This is the dominant deposition mechanism for particles in the size range 1–8 μm (as larger particles [>8 μm] are mainly deposited by inertial impaction in the proximal region of the lung).

3.3.1.3 *Brownian diffusion*

Deposition by Brownian diffusion results from the random motions of the particles caused by their collisions with surrounding gas molecules. The particle diffusion rate is proportional to the Brownian diffusion coefficient (D_B) defined as

$$D_B = \frac{CkT}{3\pi\mu d_p} \qquad (3.15)$$

where k is the Boltzmann's constant, T is the absolute temperature and C is the Cunningham correction factor. Unlike deposition by impaction and sedimentation, deposition by Brownian diffusion increases with decreasing particle size and is most efficient for particles less than 0.5 μm. A time-dependent mechanism, deposition by Brownian diffusion occurs mainly in the lung periphery (Figure 3.3). However, it should be noted that extremely small particles (less than 1 nm in diameter) are mainly filtered by the upper respiratory tract as Brownian displacements of these particles are quite high. For example, Brownian displacement in 1 s for a 1 nm particle is approximately 6 mm.

3.3.2 *Other Aerosol Deposition Mechanisms*

3.3.2.1 *Turbulent flows*

We have discussed earlier in this chapter the presence of the laryngeal jet even during quiet breathing. The laryngeal jet produces local turbulences that propagate down the bronchial tree. The flow in these regions (i.e., the upper airway and the large conducting airways) can be described in terms of a mean flow value, over which are superimposed fluctuations resulting from the local disturbances of the flow. These flow fluctuations cause particles to continuously undergo changes in their velocity both in terms of magnitude and direction. These changes can lead to particles depositing on airway walls. Deposition by turbulent mixing occurs mainly in the upper and large airways and can be as large as deposition by inertial impaction (that results from the mean flow).

3.3.2.2 *Electrostatic precipitation*

There are two types of electrostatic charges that can affect the particle transport: the space charge that refers to the repulsion between charged particles in an aerosol cloud and the image charge that refers to the attraction between a charged particle and its image charge on an electrically conducting surface. Although human airways are normally neutral, image charges with equal magnitude and opposite polarity to charged particles may be induced on the surfaces, especially inside small airways in the peripheral lung.[7] These charges generate forces that can lead to deposition by electrostatic precipitation.

3.3.2.3 *Interception*

Finally, for elongated particles such as fibers, an additional deposition mechanism needs to be considered. Deposition by interception occurs when a particle comes close enough to an airway or alveolar wall that an edge touches the surface. For example, a fiber with a length of 15 µm and a diameter of 0.4 µm has an equivalent spherical diameter of 1.5 µm, for which deposition by impaction or sedimentation is relatively low and for which interception becomes important. Deposition by interception increases with fiber length. The greater the length, the more likely the extremity of the fiber touches a surface that the center of mass would have missed.[6,8]

3.3.3 *Additional Factors Affecting Deposition*

While particle size is probably the major factor affecting particle deposition in the lung, several other factors influence not only the total deposition of particles but also their regional deposition. These factors include particle characteristics, carrier gas, physiological factors, lung anatomy and environmental factors.

3.3.3.1 *Particle characteristics*

Apart from its size, a particle is characterized by its density, shape, electrostatic charge and hygroscopic properties. Particle density affects deposition by both impaction and sedimentation but has no effect on diffusive transport. Shape can have a profound effect on the aerodynamic behavior of the particles and therefore on the deposition efficiency (see Interception). Because the relative humidity in most of the lung is near 100%, hygroscopic growth may significantly alter total and also regional deposition compared to the patterns observed with non-hygroscopic stable particles.

3.3.3.2 *Carrier gas*

In some instances, aerosol can be transported in the lung by a gas mixture other than air. The physical properties of these gases substantially affect both fluid and aerosol mechanics in the lung. Gas density affects both the pressure/flow relationship in the airways and the extent of turbulence within the flow. Helium–oxygen gas mixtures (hereafter referred to as heliox) have been used as a respiratory therapy for decades, often including aerosol.[9,10] Because of its low density, heliox flows more efficiently through constricted airways with less resistance and turbulence than air. As a consequence, deposition in the upper airway is reduced (less deposition by turbulent mixing) and a larger fraction of inhaled particles can penetrate and deposit in the more distal regions of the lung. Also, a low-density gas produces less inertial flow losses than air flow, resulting in a more uniform flow distribution especially in diseased lungs. This in turn leads to a more uniform deposition of inhaled particles.[11] Although heliox-based inhalation therapies can modify regional aerosol deposition patterns, consistent improvement in clinical outcomes has yet to be established.

3.3.3.3 *Physiological factors*

Breathing patterns, breathing frequency, tidal volume, functional residual capacity (i.e., resting lung volume), air flow dynamics and breathing pathway (oral versus nasal) all affect the extent and distribution of deposited particles in the respiratory system. Increasing air flow rates increases the efficiency of velocity-dependent deposition mechanism (impaction) and decreases that of time-dependent deposition mechanisms (sedimentation and diffusion). Increasing tidal volumes allow particles to reach more distal regions of the lung, where deposition by diffusion and sedimentation are likely to occur, therefore increasing their relative contribution to overall deposition compared to deposition by impaction. During exercise, both flow rates and tidal volumes are increased, leading to higher deposition by impaction in the large airways and by sedimentation and diffusion in the small airways and alveoli. Finally, the nasal route is more efficient at filtering particles than the oral route. Therefore, mouth breathers will tend to deposit more particles in their lungs than nose breathers.

3.3.3.4 *Anatomical factors*

Anatomical characteristics such as airway length, airway diameter, branching angles and alveolar size also play a key role in particle deposition. Because of intersubject variability, there are large variations in deposition among normal healthy subjects breathing in a similar fashion. Even within the same individual, the dimensions of the respiratory tract change with lung volume, age and pathological processes. Gender differences in lung structure also cause variations in deposition between men and women. For example, the average female thorax is smaller than in men and the volume of the conducting airways is only approximately 75% of that in men. Deposition in the tracheobronchial tree is therefore higher in women than in men. However, when these volume differences are combined with smaller resting minute ventilation and flow rates observed in women, total deposition is lower in women than in men mainly because of a smaller penetration of the aerosol in the alveolar region of the female lung.[12] Airway geometry and breathing conditions evolve from birth to adulthood. These changes affect particle deposition throughout childhood. While there are few studies on particle deposition in children, they all show that deposition in children tends to be higher than that in adults by an average factor of 1.5. More importantly, the number of particles deposited per surface area is increased by a factor 4–5 in children because of their smaller lung surface area compared to adults.

References

1. Darquenne C, Fleming JS, Katz I, Martin AR, Schroeter J, Usmani OS, Venegas J, and Schmid O. (2016). Bridging the gap between science and clinical efficacy: Physiology, imaging, and modeling of aerosols in the lung. *J. Aerosol Med. Pulm. Drug Deliv.* **29**: 107–126.
2. Bird RB, Steward WE, and Lightfoot EN. (1960). *Transport Phenomena.* New York: John Wiley & Sons, Inc.
3. Dekker E. (1961). Transition between laminar and turbulent flow in human trachea. *J. Appl. Physiol.* **16**: 1060–1064.
4. Darquenne C. (2012). Aerosol deposition in health and disease. *J Aerosol Med Pulm. Drug Deliv.* **25**: 140–147.
5. Darquenne C. (2006). Particle deposition in the lung. In: *Encyclopedia of Respiratory Medicine, Volume 3*, edited by Laurent G, and Shapiro S. Elsevier, pp. 300–304.
6. Darquenne C. (2015). Deposition of Aerosols in the Lungs: Deposition Mechanisms. In: *Textbook of Aerosol Medicine*, edited by Dhand R. Knoxville, TN: International Society for Aerosols in Medicine.

7. Kwok PCL, and Chan H-K. (2009). Electrostatics of pharmaceutical inhalation aerosols. *J. Pharm. Pharmacol.* **61**: 1587–1599.
8. Lippmann M. (1990). Effects of fiber characteristics on lung deposition, retention, and disease. *Environ. Health Perspect.* **88**: 311–317.
9. Hess DR, Fink JB, Venkataraman ST, Kim IK, Myers TR, and Tano BD. (2006). The history and physics of heliox. *Respir. Care* **51**: 608–612.
10. Kim IK, and Corcoran T. (2009). Recent developments in heliox therapy for asthma and bronchiolitis. *Clin. Pediatr. Emerg. Med.* **10**: 68–74.
11. Katz I, Pichelin M, Montesantos S, Majoral C, Martin A, Conway J, Fleming J, Venegas J, Greenblatt E, and Caillibotte G. (2014). Using helium-oxygen to improve regional deposition of inhaled particles: Mechanical principles. *J. Aerosol Med. Pulm. Drug Deliv.* **27**: 71–80.
12. Bennett WD, Zeman KL, and Kim C. (1996). Variability of fine particle deposition in healthy adults: Effect of age and gender. *Am. J. Respir. Crit. Care Med.* **153**: 1641–1647.

Chapter 4
Aerosol Measurement Techniques

4.1 Introduction

Counting and sizing of particles depends upon either capturing and characterizing the particles, which provides a degree of "ground truth" with respect to their number and properties or detecting the interaction of the particles with their environment, typically using light-based techniques.

4.2 Cascade Impactors

The reference method for counting and sizing of particles is that of the multistage cascade impactor. This is a carefully designed mechanical structure where each stage is configured in such a manner that particles with an aerodynamic diameter above a certain size are captured onto a filter or a collection cup within that stage, and where the remainder of the particles (smaller in size) remain suspended in the airstream and move to the next stage of the device. Each successive stage is configured to capture ever-decreasing particle sizes. Thus, at the end of the measurement, filters from each stage contain all particles that were in the incoming aerosol above the stage size cutoff and below the cutoff of the preceding stage.

There are several such devices in common use, but the most common are the Anderson cascade impactor and the next generation impactor (NGI). Although the geometry of each differs, they share the essential common aspects. Figure 4.1 shows the NGI and its associated geometry.

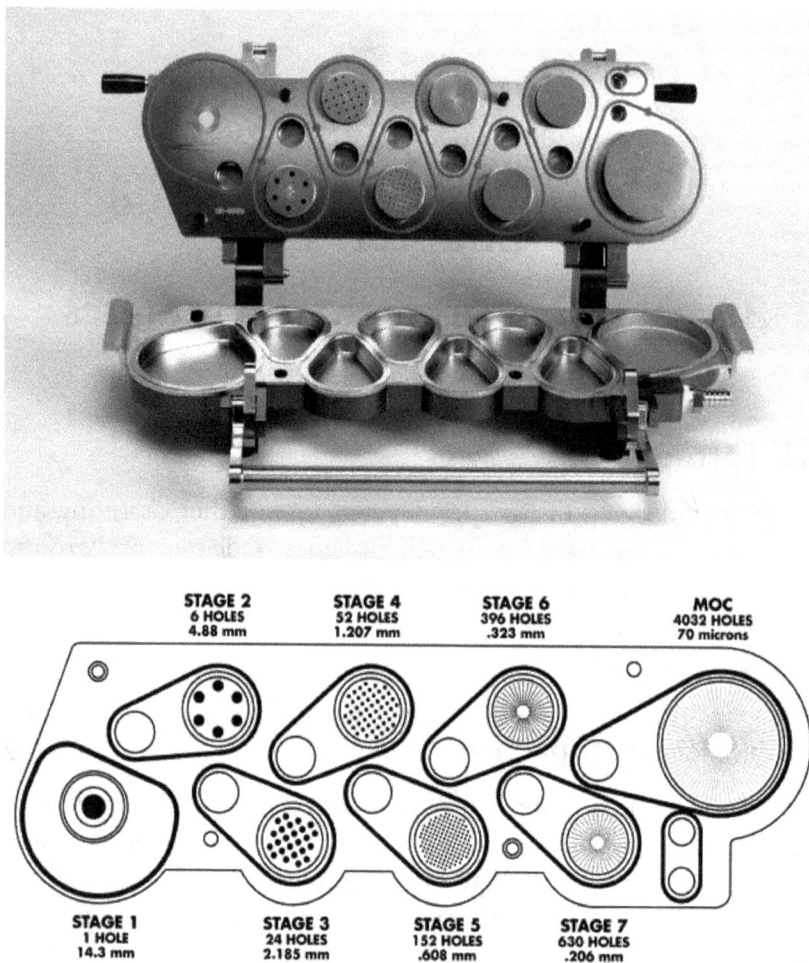

Figure 4.1: The next generation impactor (upper photo) showing the overall geometry. The lower panel shows a schematic of the entry nozzles for each stage. The air containing the particles is drawn through the system by a carefully controlled vacuum pump system via the connection point on the right. The particle-laden air enters the first (large) chamber on the left, and the largest particles impact the collection cup there. The airstream then passes to the second chamber (via a pathway in the lid) and the next range of particle sizes impact there. Note that as indicated in the lower panel, each successive stage utilizes uses an increasing number of smaller sized holes. The process continues to the micro-orifice collector (MOC) on the right (large chamber), which captures all particles smaller than those collected in the final sampling chamber. (Reproduced with permission from Copley Scientific: Quality Solutions for Inhaler Testing, 2019 edition.)

Each stage uses an impaction approach for capturing particles. Airflow enters the stage through a nozzle (a hole or series of holes) positioned directly above, but slightly separated from the collection plate or filter below it. The airflow is configured so that it is laminar with a flow rate Q. This configuration then defines the Stokes number of the incoming particles. This non-dimensional number is the ratio of the stopping distance of a particle to (in this case) the nozzle diameter. For the configuration under discussion, this is

$$St = \frac{4Q\rho_p C_c d_v^2}{9\mu\pi W^3} \qquad (4.1)$$

in which Q is the flow rate, μ is the dynamic viscosity of the carrier gas, ρ_p is the particle density, C_c is the Cunningham slip correction factor (which can reasonably be ignored for particles smaller than 2 μm), d_p is the aerodynamic diameter of the particle, and W is the nozzle diameter.

The Stokes number can be thought of as defining how "vigorously" the incoming particles enter through the nozzle, and those with higher Stokes numbers then impact (and are thus captured) on the filter or collection cup. The impactors are set up so that a value of the square root of the Stokes number above 0.49 defines the capture median value, often termed the effective cutoff diameter. Obviously, this cutoff is not perfectly sharp and so impactors define their stage efficiencies based on how broad a range of values of Stokes numbers are captured. In the NGI, the spacing between the stages is constant in logarithmic terms.

From this equation, it can be seen that the effective cutoff diameter of a stage depends on the imposed flow rate, Q. Table 4.1 provides a sample set of typical cutoff values for the 7 stages of the NGI at differing input flow rates. Of course, any given set of experiments requires careful consideration of the desired outputs as part of the experimental design, and using a cascade impactor highlights this aspect. The reader is referred to more detailed descriptions of such devices to perform appropriate experimental design.[1,2]

The obvious issue with the use of cascade impactors is that the aerosol stream is in essence destroyed as it is separated, and the

Table 4.1: The cutoff diameters at different flow rates in the next generation impactor (NGI). As flow rates are increased, only smaller particles avoid impaction in a particular stage of the impactor. The particle sizes indicated are in μm and are for spherical particles with a specific density of 1.0 (the same as water). The differences in shape or density will alter the cutoff values. (From Copley Scientific: Quality Solutions for Inhaler Testing, 2019 edition.)

STAGE	Impactor inlet flow rate			
	15 L/min	30 L/min	60 L/min	100 L/min
1	14.10	11.76	8.06	6.12
2	8.61	6.40	4.46	3.42
3	5.39	3.99	2.82	2.18
4	3.30	2.30	1.66	1.31
5	2.08	1.36	0.94	0.72
6	1.36	0.83	0.55	0.40
7	0.98	0.54	0.34	0.24
MOC	0.70	0.36	0.14	0.07

process is clearly labor-intensive with the need for careful measurement of the particle yield on each stage of the cascade impactor, and subsequent cleaning of the collectors. However, they provide the advantage of facilitating more extensive investigation of the aerosol in question, as the particles are captured by the device and are thus available for further analysis. Not only can the particle mass fraction and size fraction be determined, if desired detailed morphometric analysis of the particles themselves is possible. The latter can be important when dealing with particles generated through some processes that can generate particles in which the surface area to volume ratio can be large (i.e. particles that deviate from a simple spherical form). Such devices are clearly "laboratory only" in nature.

4.3 Real-Time Detection and Measurement of Particles

The alternative to physical collection and subsequent analysis afforded by cascade impactors are (mostly) light-based instruments. Here, rather than collecting the particles, a system is used where they are directed to a sampling region appropriately illuminated and their specific characteristics are determined. The obvious advantage of these characteristics is that they are essentially "real-time" measurements and can provide a continuous measurement of particle concentration and in some circumstances size distribution.

The devices in use fall into two broad categories: particle counters/sizers and light scattering devices. They differ substantially in their characteristics and capabilities, and so we will consider each category separately.

4.3.1 *Particle Counter/Sizers*

This class of device is designed to sample individual particles and determine the aerodynamic diameter of each particle. As counting statistics are accumulated over time, the device provides a measurement of the number fraction in a series of size "bins," in essence mimicking the output of a cascade impactor, without the need for post-collection analysis.

The general principle of the devices is a time-of-flight (TOF) design. The particle is accelerated by the airflow design in the system and then its transit time across a short distance is measured; larger particles experience greater drag than smaller particles, and so their TOF is longer. Thus, particles are characterized based on their aerodynamic diameter as this is the parameter that alters the drag.

Figure 4.2 shows a schematic for such a device. The aerosol is drawn into the device via a pump system and carefully split (via an inner nozzle) so that a small fraction is sampled. A higher flow coaxial sheath flow of clean air is then directed to surround the sampled aerosol flow, which serves to accelerate the particles towards an optical cavity illuminated to observe the particles. The optics is set up so that the light source is split providing two detection regions a short distance apart, and as the particle transits each of these regions, it is detected by the light scattered by the particle by a photodetector positioned off-axis (typically by 90°) from the illumination pathway. The time difference between the two detection events determines the particle TOF, and this is directly related to the aerodynamic diameter

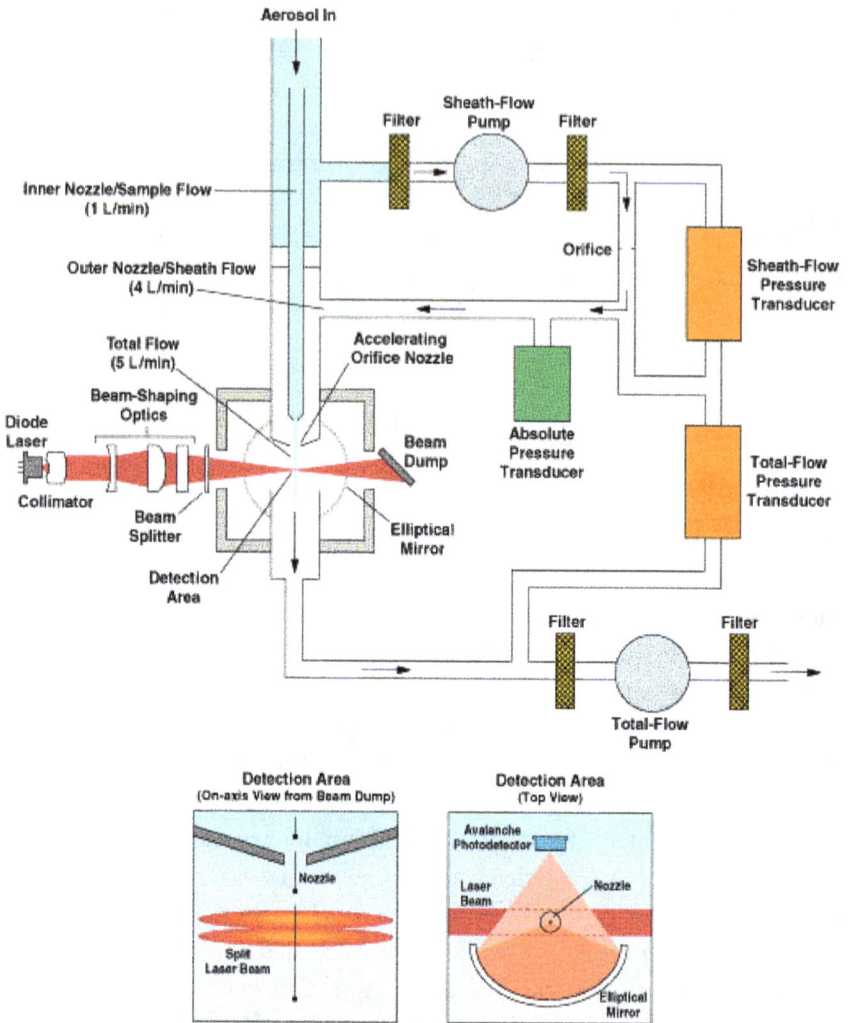

Figure 4.2:   Schematic of a time-of-flight (TOF) particle spectrometer. The aerosol is taken in and a small fraction is separated off by the inner nozzle. This is then accelerated by the sheath flow before entering the illuminated measurement region. The transit time across the split laser light source (the TOF) depends on the aerodynamic diameter of the particle. (Reproduced with permission from the International Society for Aerosols in Medicine [ISAM].)

of the particle. It should be noted however that the exact sizing assumes a number of factors that may not always be true. Typically, these include the assumption of spherical particles and particles with a density equivalent to that of water. In cases in which these conditions are not met, further calibration/characterization of the device output may be necessary.

The obvious limitation of this approach is the need to measure particles individually. The principle upon which the technique depends assumes that only a single particle is crossing the TOF region of the analyzer at any one time, and it is easy to imagine that the simultaneous presence of two particles in the sampling region (perhaps two particles of differing sizes) leads to ambiguities in the timing intervals upon which the TOF measurement depends. This has the potential to mischaracterize the sizes of these particles. The modern devices however have high sampling rates (up to 100,000 particles/min), which serve to allow the sampling of higher aerosol concentrations.

While the algorithms used in the systems are sophisticated enough to generally discount data from coincidence counting events, in order to work effectively, there needs to be a reasonable expectation that a good proportion of the events are indeed single particle in nature. This necessitates careful consideration of the input aerosol number density and this is partly accomplished by having only a portion of the sampled aerosol stream be sent for analysis (typically ~20%) and if required by using one or two diluter modules in front of the sampling system to dilute the sampled aerosol. The diluters themselves are variations in the sampling system shown in Figure 4.2, where the incoming aerosol flow is split and a higher volume, aerosol-free, sheath flow is combined with it, diluting the incoming concentration. Typical dilution ratios are 20:1 and 100:1, and so by using two such devices in series, dilutions of up to 10,000:1 are possible.

These counter/sizer devices all require sampling of the aerosol source as they all work by drawing the aerosol into the sampling system, unlike cascade impactors in which often the entire aerosol source can be sampled. Thus, it is important to consider how the aerosol is sampled from its source. There are no universal rules for how such sampling should be done, as in general it is highly configuration-specific, but care and forethought must be employed to ensure that the sample drawn from the experiment is indeed representative of the overall aerosol source. In short, there is no substitute for good experimental design.

The advantages of aerosol sizers over cascade impactors are the obvious ones of speed of analysis and the absence of the need to clean the device between every experiment. Further, the resolution of the sampled size distribution (the "bin" width of the device) is very much higher (by an order of magnitude) than cascade impactors, with resolutions of 0.02–0.03 µm possible.

Alternatives to the detection by TOF light systems exist, such as approaches in which the relaxation of particle oscillations induced by either acoustic waves or alternating electric fields has been used. However, the factor in common across all such methods is the need to measure particles individually, and this brings with it the need to limit particle concentrations and/or the use of diluters as described above. Further, some experimental studies have used mass spectrometry to characterize particles immediately after they have been measured in a TOF system.[3]

4.4 Light Scattering Devices

While both cascade impactors and particle sizers collect or sample the aerosol, light scattering devices can be configured to simply "observe" the aerosol. This can be advantageous in some circumstances such as human or animal experimentation as the inhaled or exhaled aerosol can be measured as it travels unimpeded.

Light scattering devices are not new and simple versions date back many decades. Early versions such as the tyndallometer, named after John Tyndall who provided early work on the scattering of light, were a light source with scattered light detection at 90° from the incident direction.[4] Later versions use a laser source, typically He-Ne, providing monochromatic light in the red part of the spectrum (632.8 nm). Using high-angle scattering results in a simple linear instrument that provides a signal proportional to the number of particles in the illuminated region, which is essentially a measure of the particle concentration. However, the limitation in such a device is that the particles in question need to be of the same size since the intensity of the scattered light is dependent on particle size. Hence the use of such devices is limited to work with monodisperse particles. Nevertheless, much use can be made of such devices in some studies.[5,6]

More sophisticated devices utilize low-angle light scattering. In order for this to work, a monochromatic coherent light is required (i.e., a laser source) and such devices fall under the category of laser diffractometry. Again He-Ne lasers are a common source. The technique utilizes Fraunhofer scattering in which incident light is forward-scattered (i.e. scattered in the same general direction as the incident light source) and produces a series of concentric rings around the incident axis. For a small spherical particle, these rings are widely separated, but are closer together as the particle size increases (Figure 4.3).

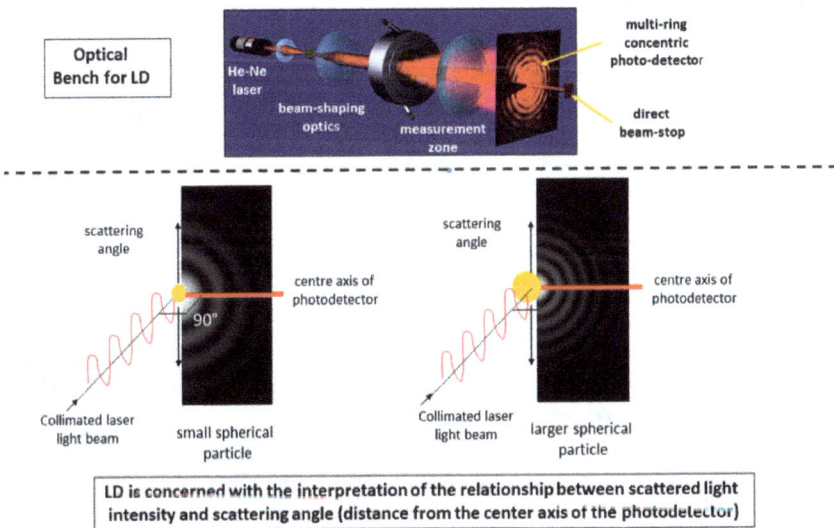

Figure 4.3: Low-angle forward light scattering by particles of different sizes. The forward-scattered light forms concentric interference rings around the axis of the incident light source. The smaller the particle, the greater the wavelength of the interference rings. (Reproduced with permission from the International Society for Aerosols in Medicine [ISAM].)

The detectors are arranged such that the diffraction rings can be determined. Rather than measuring the characteristic of a single particle as in the TOF devices, these instruments can determine the volume-weighted size distribution of all the particles present in the measurement zone at a point in time. Modern devices have very high sampling rates of up to 2500 samples per second. Devices can be based on either the Fraunhofer theory (applicable for spherical particles much larger than the wavelength of the light) or the more complete Lorenz-Mie model. However, as for any technique, care must be utilized in cases in which particle geometry (in particular) deviates from that in the underlying theory. Nevertheless, sizing distributions from sub-micron to hundreds of microns are possible, although changes in external optics are generally required to cover the full range of possible sizes.

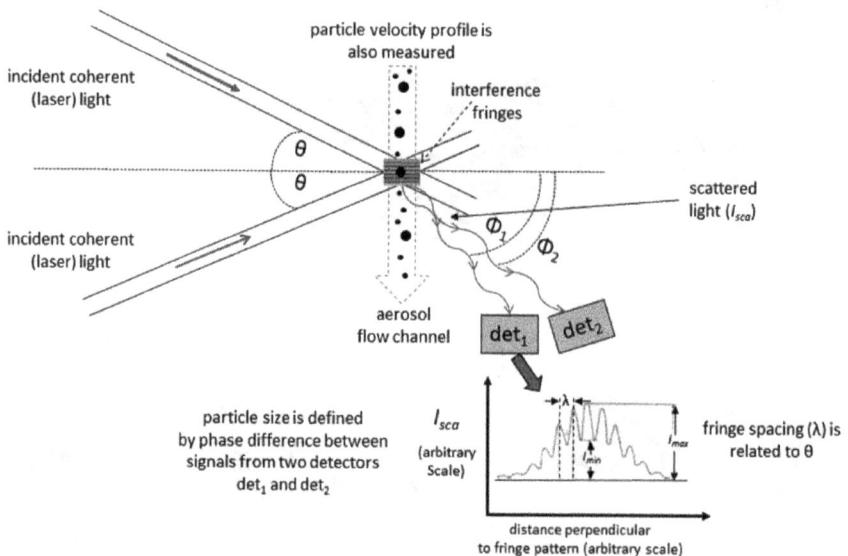

Figure 4.4: Schematic describing the principle upon which laser-phase Doppler anemometry is based. The two intersecting lasers produce an interference pattern in the measurement zone. As the particle being measured transits the measurement zone, it scatters light, which results in two Doppler busts, measured by two detectors positioned at different angular locations. (Reproduced with permission from the International Society for Aerosols in Medicine [ISAM].)

Other optical technologies can also be employed. Laser-phase Doppler anemometry is a technique in which a particle's transit across the measurement field is determined. This field is illuminated by beams from two coherent light sources that cross each other. These two light beams establish a series of interference fringes where they cross. As the particle transits this field, two Doppler bursts are detected at slightly different angular positions and the phase difference between them determined.[7] Once again, there are intrinsic assumptions that are implicit (in particular, particle geometry, which is assumed to be spherical), which must be taken into consideration. The technique also provides a measurement of particle velocity, making it useful in situations such as measuring the plumes emitted by devices such as pressurized metered-dose inhalers.

A brief summary of the various approaches to particle size measurement is presented in Table 4.2.

Table 4.2:   Approaches to the measurement of particles size and concentration.

Device	Principle	Size determination	Size range	Real time
Cascade Impactor	Impaction	Yes Considered the "gold standard" technique	Wide: 14 to less than 1 µm	No
Time of Flight (TOF)	Particle acceleration	Yes	Wide ranges: 20 µm to sub-micron ranges possible	Yes. Dilution often required
Tyndallometer	Side scattering of light Bulk aerosol determination	No	Wide but aerosol must be mono-disperse	Yes
Laser Diffractometry	Forward scattering of coherent light	Yes	Limited to large spherical particles (>~25 µm)	Yes
Laser-Phase Doppler Anemometer	Light scatters as particle transits interference fringes	Yes Velocity also determined	Very wide: 0.3 to 8000 µm	Yes

References

1. Marple VA, Roberts DL, Romay FJ, Miller NC, Truman KG, Van Oort M, Olsson B, Holroyd MJ, Mitchell JP, and Hochrainer D. (2003). Next generation pharmaceutical impactor (a new impactor for pharmaceutical inhaler testing). Part I: Design. *J. Aerosol Med.* **16:** 283–299.
2. Marple VA, Olson BA, Santhanakrishnan K, Mitchell JP, Murray SC, and Hudson-Curtis BL. (2003). Next generation pharmaceutical impactor (a new impactor for pharmaceutical inhaler testing). Part II: Archival calibration. *J. Aerosol Med.* **16:** 301–324.
3. Fergenson DP, Pitesky ME, Tobias HJ, *et al.* (2004). Reagentless detection and classification of individual bioaerosol particles in seconds. *Anal. Chem.* **76:** 373–378.
4. Hoffman RA, and Billingham J. (1975). Effect of altered G levels on deposition of particulates in the human respiratory tract. *J. Appl. Physiol.* **38:** 955–960.
5. Darquenne C, Paiva M, West JB, and Prisk GK. (1997). Effect of microgravity and hypergravity on deposition of 0.5- to 3-μm-diameter aerosol in the human lung. *J. Appl. Physiol.* **83:** 2029–2036.
6. Darquenne C, West JB, and Prisk GK. (1998). Deposition and dispersion of 1 μm aerosol boluses in the human lung: Effect of micro- and hypergravity. *J. Appl. Physiol.* **85:** 1252–1259.
7. Stapleton KW, Finlay WH, and Zuberbuhler P. (1994). An in vitro method for determining regional dosages delivered by jet nebulizers. *J. Aerosol Med.* **7:** 325–344.

Chapter 5
Determination of Aerosol Deposition

5.1 Experimental Determination of Aerosol Deposition

This section provides a brief overview of how measurements of aerosol deposition are made with a deliberate emphasis on techniques used in humans. In general, the same techniques may be applicable in animal studies, although it is often far from trivial to take a measurement technique and scale it down to a size suitable for use in small animal studies, while still maintaining adequate accuracy and sensitivity.

5.1.1 *Measuring Total Deposition*

Measurement of total deposition is essentially a process of measuring the difference between the amount of aerosol inhaled and the amount subsequently exhaled, with the assumption that the difference must reflect that deposited. Like any experiment of this nature, the choice of measurement technique depends on the ability to accurately and reproducibly perform the inhaled and exhaled measurements, and errors associated with the chosen measurement techniques also need to be considered.

A schematic of a basic experiment is shown in Figure 5.1.

In this configuration, the system was designed to determine the deposition of a monodisperse aerosol. The use of a monodisperse particle source is necessary since the use of a photometer (near the

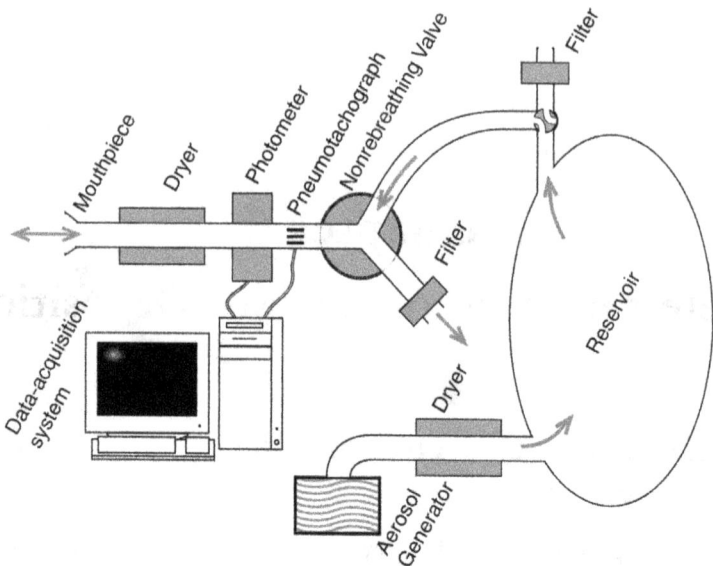

Figure 5.1: The basic setup of a system for the measurement of total aerosol deposition in humans. The salient features of the system are discussed in the text. Used with permission from Ref. 1.

mouthpiece) depends on scattered light, and the amount of scattering depends on particle size (see Chapter 4). Thus, a quantitative measurement of particle concentration requires that all particles should be of the same size (monodisperse). Although one could imagine using a particles sizer/counter in place of the (much simpler) photometer, obviating the need for a monodisperse aerosol, such a device would need to be capable of very high throughput rates to cope with the typical breathing frequencies involved (where inspiration and expiration might each last only ~2 s).

The aerosol is generated and, because in this case, a solid particle was used (polystyrene latex particles), dried before being delivered to a large reservoir (a large Mylar coated Douglas bag). The reservoir provided a means by which the rate of aerosol generation could differ from the rate of delivery to the subject. This system provides a large volume of dry, monodisperse aerosol, which could then be used for measurements of total deposition, whenever the experiment is performed. While there is some loss of aerosol in the reservoir bag due to sedimentation, the dimensions of the bag are sufficiently large (tens of cm and more) that the loss is minimal provided the experiments are performed within a few minutes of aerosol generation.

The key aspects of the actual measurement system are shown in the upper left quadrant of Figure 5.1. The photometer is located close to the mouthpiece (and most importantly, before any other devices and valves) to ensure that the aerosol concentration measured is as close as possible to that entering the subject's mouth. The dryer placed between the photometer and mouthpiece is of a co-axial design where the drying agent surrounds an otherwise unobstructed tube. This dryer is required because the exhaled particles will likely have acquired a coating of water during their time in the respiratory tract in saturated air and so will have increased in size slightly, thereby generating an increased signal detected by the photometer. Therefore, it is necessary to dry the aerosol before measuring the concentration (recall that the aerosol contained in the reservoir was already dry).

Beyond the photometer, the pneumotachograph (flowmeter) measures the respired volume of the subject. A non-rebreathing valve (NRV) allows for inspiration from either room air or from the reservoir bag (depending on the position of the valve just above the reservoir). Both the pneumotachograph and the valves will cause a degree of aerosol deposition to occur in these parts of the plumbing system, but because the photometer is located on the subject side of these devices, losses here do not affect the measurement.

Figure 5.2 shows a typical trace from the device shown in Figure 5.1. Note that because aerosols deposit in the lung as opposed to mixing with gas contained within the lung, a steady-state condition is reached after only about 1 breath (in contrast to gas mixing, which takes many breaths to reach steady state because the gas must mix with the substantial amount of air in the lung at end-expiration). It can be seen that there is steady concentration of inspired aerosol (consistent with the use of the reservoir) and that the expired concentration of aerosol is very much lower than inspired concentration as a result of deposition in the lung.

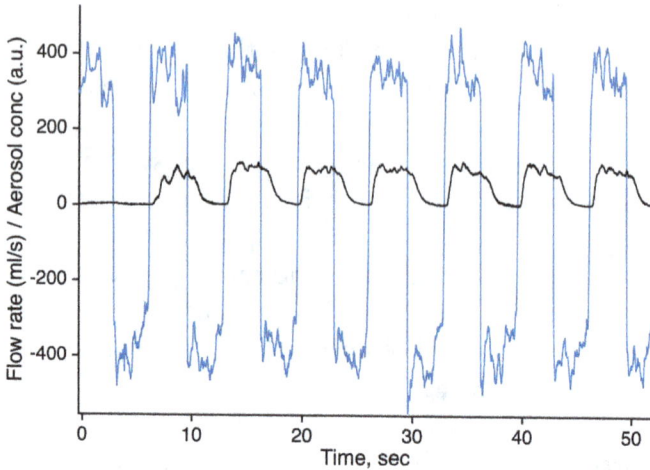

Figure 5.2:   A typical experimental trace from the system like that shown in Figure 5.1. Aerosol concentration is shown in black, and the flow is shown in blue (inspiration is positive). It can be readily appreciated that the expired aerosol concentration rapidly achieves a steady state soon after the beginning of expiration.

Deposition is calculated from the following equation:

$$DE = 1 - N_{ex}/N_{in} \times V_{in}/V_{ex} \qquad (5.1)$$

where N is the number of particles inspired (in) or expired (ex) in a breath (essentially the integral of the zero-baseline-corrected photometer signal over the period of interest), and V is the corresponding volume of the breath (from integration of the flow signal from the pneumotachograph). In order to perform these integrations with accuracy, it is necessary to have a sufficiently high data sampling rate to accurately characterize both the flow and the aerosol concentration profile. For the system described above, a sampling rate of 100 Hz is used, which, given a typical inspiratory or expiratory time of ~2 s, is more than adequate. If one is to consider steady-state deposition, then it is important to consider only breaths in which V_{in} and V_{ex} are the same (to within some predetermined tolerance), as without this step, a larger or smaller V_{ex} than V_{in} would result in more or fewer particles being exhaled than those that remain suspended in the airways.

   Clearly, there are other possible experimental designs that could be used to measure total deposition of inhaled aerosol. However, the description above should serve to highlight the salient features of the process. Changes in any of the components or design elements are certainly possible but require cognizance of the potential pitfalls of the altered technology and how these changes might affect the measurement.

5.1.2 *Bolus Deposition*

While the measurement of total deposition described in Section 5.1.1 is a useful and often necessary measurement, it fails to provide any information about the mechanism or site of deposition. A more informative approach is the bolus technique that allows the investigator to gain information into the site and nature of the processes that occur. In a bolus experiment, instead of an aerosol being delivered in a continuous fashion throughout inspiration, a small volume of aerosol laden air (a bolus) is delivered at a specific point in an inspiration. When the bolus is delivered therefore determines how deep into the lung the aerosol reaches. If a bolus is delivered early in inspiration, it traverses the central airways and reaches the lung periphery. In contrast, if a bolus is delivered very late in the inspiration, then it may only reach the central airways. It is this ability to probe different "depths" within a breath that is useful.

Following on from the previous section, Figure 5.3 shows a bolus delivery and measurement system. In this case, the data acquisition system and the components close to the subject are the same as those used in the total deposition studies. However, the aerosol preparation and holding system differ. Rather than a large reservoir bag (Figure 5.1), the aerosol is generated, dried, and delivered to a tube of known volume, that region between SV2 and SV3, termed the Bolus Tube. While this occurs, the subject breathes filtered air through the valve SV1 and the NRV.

The test is usually initiated by having the subject predetermine his or her lung volume, either residual volume (RV, the lowest possible lung volume) or functional residual capacity (FRC, the end of a normal passive expiration). The subject then begins a test inspiration of a preplanned volume, and after an appropriate volume is inspired, the solenoid valves SV1 and SV3 are switched so that the inspiratory path

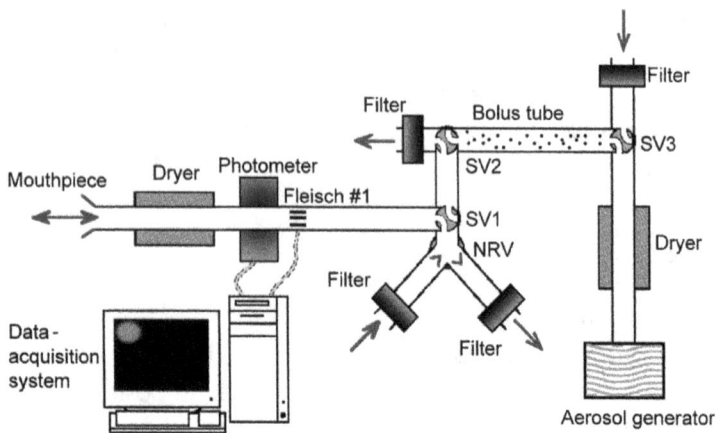

Figure 5.3: A typical experimental configuration for an aerosol bolus study. The measurement system is that in Figure 5.1 used for total deposition studies, but the aerosol delivery system is modified. See text for details. Used with permission from Ref. 2.

is via the bolus tube. Inspiration continues until the preplanned inspiratory volume is reached at which time SV2 switches, preventing further inspiration and the subject then exhales via SV1 and SV2. The volume of air from the start of the aerosol inhalation to the end of the preplanned inspiration is termed the penetration volume of the test (V_p).

From this description, it can be seen that if the initial valve switch occurs very early in the preplanned inspiration, then V_p will be large and the bolus will reach the lung periphery. In contrast, if the switch occurs late in the inspiration, V_p will be low and the bolus will only reach the central airways. To improve reproducibility of the tests, it is usual to standardize the timing by having the subjects inspire and expire at a fixed flow rate by providing them with a visual feedback of the respired flow rate.

Figure 5.4A shows a tracing of such a test. Zero volume represents the volume at end inspiration. Inspiration began 2 L below this volume (at either RV or FRC), and at 500 mL before the end of the 2-L test inspiration, the bolus was inspired. The bolus can be seen to be quite narrow (the bolus tube contains only 70 mL) and once the

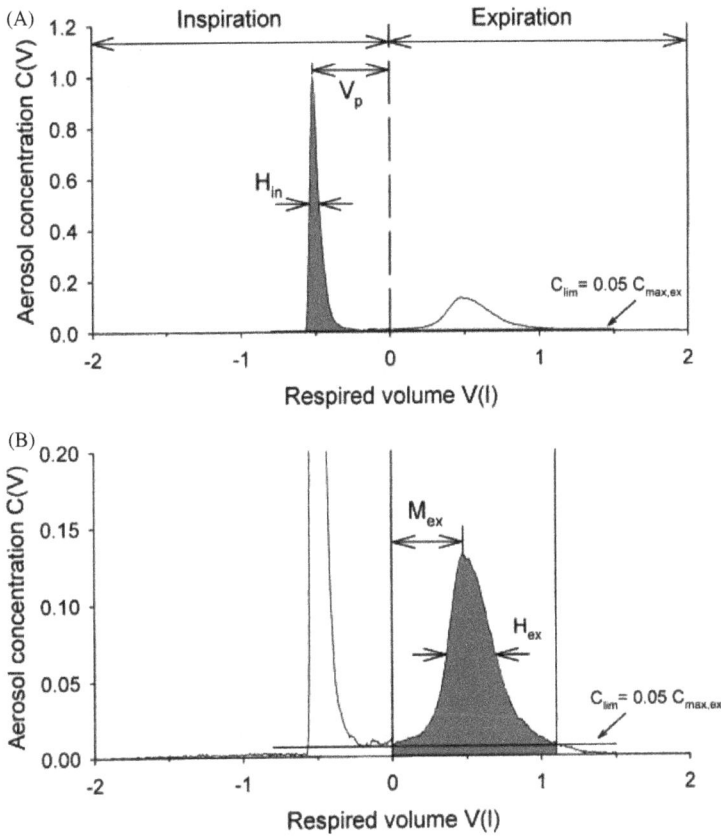

Figure 5.4: A typical trace from an aerosol bolus study. The vertical axis displays aerosol concentration, while the horizontal axis is a time axis that is labeled to show respired volume. The details are provided in the text. Used with permission from Ref. 2.

bolus is inspired, the remaining part of the inspiration is aerosol-free gas. Once the target inspired volume is reached (and the valve moves, preventing further inspiration), the subject expires, again at a constant flow rate to the starting lung volume of the test. During this expiration, it can be seen that there is an exhaled bolus, centered at approximately the same expired volume as the V_p (in this case, 500 mL, but variation in the peak of the bolus occurs and is termed mode shift) and the peak is "tilted" to the left (skew). The expired bolus is wider than the inspired bolus (termed dispersion). Further, the area under the expired bolus is less than that under the inspired bolus due to aerosol deposition. The calculation and utility of bolus deposition, dispersion, and mode shift are discussed in the sections that follow.

5.1.2.1 *Deposition*

The calculation of bolus deposition is essentially the same as that of total deposition (Eq. (5.1)) applied over the single test inspiration/expiration. However, because the inspiratory and expiratory volumes are so tightly controlled, this reduces to

$$De = 1 - N_{ex}/N_{in} \qquad (5.2)$$

An important point here is that it is necessary to consider only data in which the aerosol signal exceeds a predefined threshold in order for the measurement not to be contaminated by the inevitable presence of noise in the photometer signal. This threshold depends on the intrinsic noise of the system, but for the example shown in Figure 5.4, the threshold was set at 5% of the maximum concentration observed in the expired bolus signal. This eliminates only a very small amount of signal and greatly improves data reliability.

Typical results are shown in Figure 5.5A, which shows deposition values for three particle sizes and penetration volumes (V_p) between 200 and 1500 mL in four normal subjects. As expected, deposition is generally higher for larger particles sizes, an effect expected because the rate of gravitational sedimentation is higher for the more massive, large particles. Deposition also increases as penetration volume increases, which is of course an inevitable result because a bolus inspired deep into the lung must necessarily traverse the central airways, and so experiences the same deposition losses as a shallowly inspired bolus experience along its travel path. However, it can also be seen that the rate at which deposition rises with penetration volume is also particle size-dependent, with more massive particles accumulating deposition more rapidly than smaller particles. This is again due to the effect of gravitational sedimentation; when the same studies are performed in the absence of gravity (see Chapter 11),

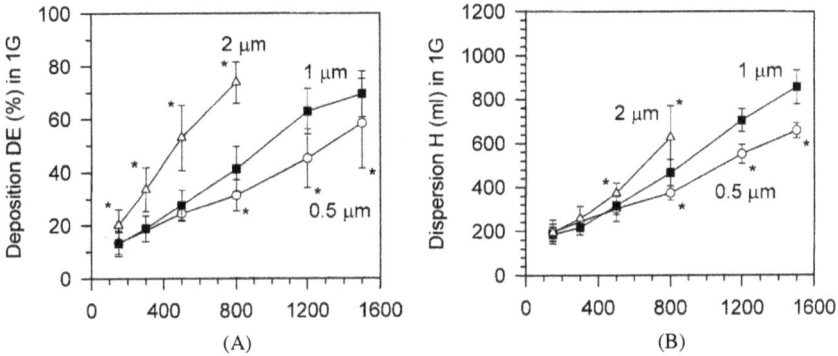

Figure 5.5: Left panel: Deposition as a function of penetration volume for three different particle sizes. The details are explained in the text. Note that as particle size increases, so too does deposition, consistent with increased gravitational sedimentation of the more massive particles. Right panel: Dispersion as a function of penetration volume at three different particles sizes in the same subject as in the left panel. Used with permission from Ref. 3.

deposition as a function of penetration volume is completely independent of particle size between 0.5 and 2 μm.[3] Notably, for the largest particles studied (2 μm), penetration volumes above 800 mL had essentially 100% deposition, resulting in the absence of an expired bolus signal.

5.1.2.2 *Dispersion*

Dispersion is the degree to which the expired bolus is wider than the inspired bolus. This widening is a direct reflection of the degree of heterogeneity in the flow within the lung and heterogeneity of the pathways within the lung. In essence, a bolus experiment measuring dispersion looks at how convective mixing in the lung serves to make a bolus "spread-out" in its travel path into and out of the bronchial tree. The aerosol bolus can be considered as a "non-diffusing gas", thus allowing convective processes to be studied without the ever-present effects of diffusion that are present when an actual gas is used. In short, the aerosol bolus dispersion is a measurement of the total amount of mixing that the particles have undergone and thus is expected to increase when ventilation to different regions of the lung is uneven, and there is a difference in the sequence of filling and emptying of these regions. Such heterogeneity in ventilation and asynchronous flow is present in all lungs and typically increases in the presence of disease.

Dispersion is calculated as the increase in half-width of the expired bolus compared to the inspired bolus. The half-width is defined as the bolus width (in ml) between the two points at one half of the maximum concentration of the bolus (see Figure 5.4B). Having defined the widths of the inspired and expired boluses (H_{in} and H_{ex}, respectively), Dispersion (also in mL) is defined as

$$H = (H_{ex}^2 - H_{in}^2)^{1/2} \tag{5.3}$$

As with deposition, dispersion (Figure 5.5, right panel) increases with penetration volume, an expected result, as the bolus must traverse more branch points in the bronchial tree in cases of larger V_p. However, unlike deposition, the differences in dispersion as a function of particles size are comparatively small, with all three particle sizes studied providing indistinguishable results for shallow penetration volumes. At higher penetration volumes, there is a modest increase in dispersion as particle size increases. It becomes apparent that this is a direct consequence of increased sedimentation with larger particles; when the same measurements are performed in the absence of gravity, dispersion is essentially identical for all three sizes, although it of course increased with increasing penetration volume (see Chapter 11). The results indicate that provided sedimentation is controlled for (i.e. a single particle size is used), dispersion can usefully be employed as a measure of convective heterogeneity of pulmonary ventilation.

5.1.2.3 *Mode shift*

As the bolus traverses the bronchial tree, there is also a tendency for the mode (the peak of the bolus) to alter in its volumetric position. This is termed mode shift. It is defined by the following equation:

$$MS = M_{ex} - V_p \tag{5.4}$$

where the term M_{ex} is the volumetric position of the peak of the exhaled bolus relative to the end-inspiratory volume (see Figure 5.4). As a general rule, mode shift is close to zero for shallow penetration volumes and becomes progressively more negative (i.e. the expired bolus appears earlier in expiration that would be expected based on the penetration volume) as V_p and particles size increase.[3] As is the case with both deposition and dispersion, the changes in mode shift with particle size disappear in the absence of gravity, indicating that they are a consequence of the sedimentation rate of the particles. It is thought that the basis of the mode shift increase with increased sedimentation is that the portion of the inspired bolus that penetrates most deeply into the lung experiences greater sedimentary loss than the more shallowly inhaled portions of the bolus, and this results in the distal part of the bolus being "pruned" with an attendant shift in the peak of the exhaled bolus towards shallower penetration volumes.

Little use can be made of the mode shift as a probe into lung function. It is difficult to accurately measure and is thus relatively poorly understood. One study[4] used changes in posture to induce changes in flow sequencing in the lung (the order in which different lung units empty). The supine posture is associated with increased flow sequencing, and when the mode shift of 0.5 μm boluses was measured, there was a slightly more mouthward change in the mode shift at all penetration volumes that was strongly associated with the degree of flow sequencing inferred from gas washout tests. It should, however, be emphasized that the effects seen were rather small and this is unlikely to be a clinically useful tool.

5.2 Imaging

While much can be inferred from aerosol studies that utilize inspired and expired measurements (Section 5.1), all these approaches suffer from the same problem; they provide no spatial information of processes that are clearly distributed throughout the lung. In many cases, the question of where aerosol deposits may be equally as important as how much of that aerosol deposits. In order to address questions that have a spatial component, a form of spatial measurement is required. This section briefly introduces some of the techniques available for such studies, although for the details of such methods the reader is referred to more specialized texts.

In terms of imaging inhaled aerosols and where they deposit in the lung, some form of tracer or contrast agent to identify the aerosol is required. The aerosol particles themselves do not generally generate a signal that is detectable by standard imaging systems and so some labeling is needed. This labeling takes the form of attaching a radioactive tracer or fluorescent marker to the particles or of adding a contrast agent to the particles appropriate for the imaging modality being used. In some cases, the particles themselves can be directly imaged, typically based on their magnetic properties.

5.2.1 *Planar Gamma Scintigraphy*

The most common form of imaging employed with inhaled aerosols is planar gamma scintigraphy in which the spatial location of particle deposition is measured in a two-dimensional (2D) plane using what is commonly called a gamma camera.

As the name suggests, this imaging modality uses the emission of high energy photons (gamma radiation) from particles that have been labeled with a gamma emitter. The most common tracer used is ^{99m}Tc (metastable Technicium-99), which emits photons with an energy of 140 KeV and decays with a half-life of 6.01 h. Other tracers are used in certain circumstances and these have different half-lives and emission energies. Dual tracer studies using different energies can be performed in some circumstances as the gamma camera can detect the energy of the photons it sees. In a typical experiment, a labeled material is aerosolized, inhaled by the subject, and deposited in the lung; the subject is then imaged.

Figure 5.6 provides a brief overview of a planar gamma scintigraphy system. The camera head is typically mounted on a gantry to allow it to be brought into close proximity to the region being imaged. For lung imaging, this typically means having the subject supine with the camera head placed in close proximity to the anterior

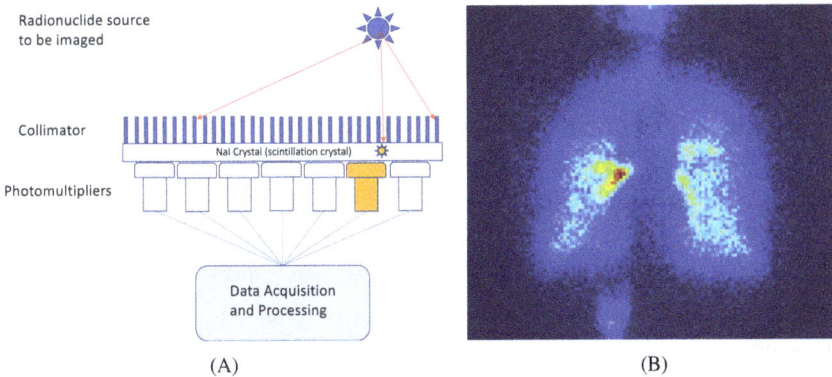

Figure 5.6: (A) Top-level schematic of a gamma camera, (B) An image of aerosol deposition in the lung from such a device.

chest wall or having the camera be the "back of the chair" and having the subject sit in front of it.

The photons emitted from the deposited tracer are emitted in all directions and so the front of the gamma camera consists of a collimator, i.e. a photon absorbing plate through which there is a series of perpendicular holes arranged in a grid. Because these holes are typically deeper than their diameter, they serve to allow only photons that are emitted along their axis to pass through, and so it can be thought of as ensuring that the gamma camera only "looks" at a region directly in front of it. Thus, photons that are emitted at an angle that is not close to 90° from the face of the camera are filtered out.

Photons that pass through the collimator unimpeded then hit a large scintillation crystal (typically sodium iodide, NaI) that emits a flash of light when the gamma photon is absorbed. The intensity of the flash depends on the energy of the photon absorbed. Immediately behind the scintillation crystal is an array of photomultiplier tubes (PMTs), optically coupled to the crystal. These devices convert a flash of light into an electrical signal and this is collected by the data acquisition system. The front faces of the PMTs are typically quite large (a diameter of ~100 mm is common), but the flash of light will be registered by multiple adjacent PMTs, which enables the estimation of the spatial position of registered photons.

It is important to recognize that an image from planar gamma scintigraphy is an image from all sources that are in front of the collimator without regard to their distance from the collimator. A pixel in the image in Figure 5.6B could have resulted from a point in the anterior lung or the posterior lung. This type of image is termed a "projection image" and is in essence the integration of all activity along the through-plane axis of the 2D image.

The in-plane spatial resolution of a gamma camera image is a complex amalgam of several factors. The energy of the emitted gamma photon results in a different degree of scattering within the tissues of the body. Two images acquired with different energy tracers will have somewhat different spatial resolutions. The distance from the point of emission to the collimator affects resolution with points closer to the collimator being better located than those far away. Thus, in a projection image, there is a combination of resolutions that depend on the through-plane distances involved. The properties of the collimator alter spatial resolution and manufacturers produce different collimators for different imaging applications. The properties of the PMT array and electronics all contribute to overall resolution. As such, there is no way to specify a particular resolution for a device without being cognizant of these factors and likely performing some calibration studies.

There is a final point that must be considered when considering resolution and this is imaging time. In order to limit the dose of ionizing radiation to the subject (a critically important issue in all human studies), imaging needs to be performed with the lowest possible dose of tracer, limiting the number of photons available for detection. In order to obtain adequate counting statistics from the gamma camera, image acquisition times are therefore long (typically the order of several minutes). This means then that the subject must be breathing during the image acquisition and so the images acquired include a degree of motion artifact, especially when considering lung images. Because most of the motion of the lung during quiet breathing is near the diaphragm, this effect is typically greater in the basal lung regions. Further, as imaging times increase the ability of a subject to remain motionless with respect to the camera becomes less, further adding motion artifact. Overall, however, the spatial resolution (the ability to resolve 2 point sources) of a planar gamma scintigraph of the lung is of the order of a ~1–2 cm in size. Further, the choice of tracer employed serves to alter the degree of scattering of photons by the overlying issue. As different tracers have different energies of the emitted photons, they are scattered differently, with the effect being that the degradation in resolution differs. Further, the labeling of a drug to be imaged must be carefully performed in order that the addition of the radiotracer does not alter the aerodynamic properties of the inhaled substance.[5]

There are multiple means of analyzing planar scintigraphy images, and just a few simple overviews are described here. As with any image-based technique, there is generally some need to extract some numerical values for statistical comparison. The simplest of these are based on an analysis of the histogram of the lung region of interest image. As the deposition of the tracer (and hence, the activity detected in the planar image) is taken as a marker of ventilation, only computing the width of the histogram of activity, typically by using the second moment or standard deviation, provides a useful measure of heterogeneity. Figure 5.7 shows a typical set of images. Further, the third moment or skew of the distribution has been shown to be a useful measure, as this increases in the face of higher spatial heterogeneity, especially in the presence of "hot spots," such as might be seen in regions of high deposition in airways.[6]

While analysis of the distribution of deposition is useful, it serves to eliminate any actual spatial information contained in the images, and in doing so, eliminates potentially useful information. The central-to-peripheral ratio of lung activity provides a simple means of moving into a description of spatial information and is illustrated in Figure 5.7. The technique is relatively simple to implement.

While the basic analysis of planar images can be reasonably simply described, when it comes to other three-dimensional (3D) imaging techniques described in the following sections, the variety of analysis techniques employed is almost as varied as the number of studies performed. As such, it is impractical to provide a general overview of those techniques, and they need to be examined within the context of the individual studies.

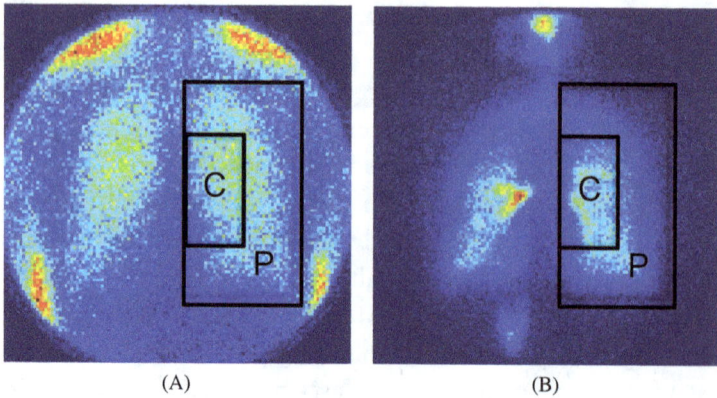

(A)   (B)

Figure 5.7:   Transmission scan (A) and deposition scan (B) of ^{99m}Tc aerosol. The transmission scan produced using a ^{57}Co planar source in front of the subject is used to define the limits of the right lung extent in the superior/inferior and left-right directions. The rectangular box is then divided into a central region covering half of the vertical and horizontal extent of the lung, positioned centrally in the vertical dimension and medially in the horizontal direction, with the remainder being classed as peripheral. The activity can then be expressed as the C/P ratio, where a uniform deposition would result in a value near 1.0. The C/P ratio of the deposition scan is ~1.4 in this example, indicating greater deposition in the central airways. Modified from Ref. 7.

5.2.2 *SPECT*

Single-photon emission computed tomography (SPECT) is an extension of planar gamma scintigraphy to 3D. The process of obtaining 3D information from a 2D measurement system is entirely analogous to the manner in which 2D planar X-ray images, taken from multiple angles, can be combined to form a cross-sectional image of the body, i.e. computed tomography (CT). A SPECT acquisition system works by taking a series of 2D projection images using a planar gamma scintigraphy system (see Section 5.2.1) with each image taken in a different rotational position around the object being imaged. A typical system is shown in Figure 5.8.

Because SPECT requires multiple images, the imaging times can often be longer than planar imaging. To keep imaging times reasonable, a higher dose of tracer can be used, but this of course comes with a higher dose of ionizing radiation to the patient. Nevertheless, the improved spatial information may be useful, particularly in

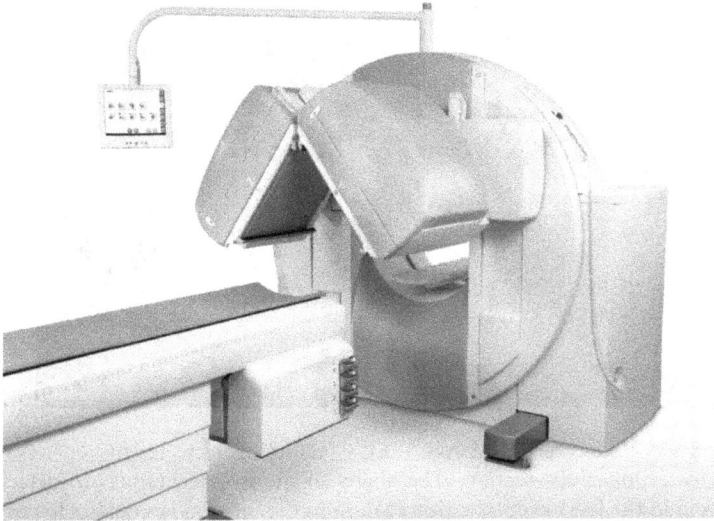

Figure 5.8: A SPECT imaging system. In this system, two planar gamma cameras are rotated around the subject and the series of projection images from different angles are combined into a 3D volume image.

clinical studies. Figure 5.9 shows a SPECT image superimposed over an anatomical X-ray CT image. For comparison, the comparable positron emission tomography (PET) image is also provided (see also Section 5.2.3).

5.2.3 *PET — Coincidence Counting*

Positron Emission Tomography (PET) differs from other radioactive tracer techniques that it uses coincidence counting to improve the spatial resolution of the images. In PET, the tracers used are positron emitters (a positron is the antimatter equivalent of an electron). As soon as the positron is emitted by the radioactive decay process, it rapidly encounters a nearby electron and both are annihilated, resulting in the emission of two 0.511 MeV photons traveling in opposite directions (a result of conservation of momentum; Figure 5.10). The PET scanner consists of one or more rings of detectors, and when two detectors across the ring register simultaneous events, the point of decay must be along the line connecting those two detectors. This so-called

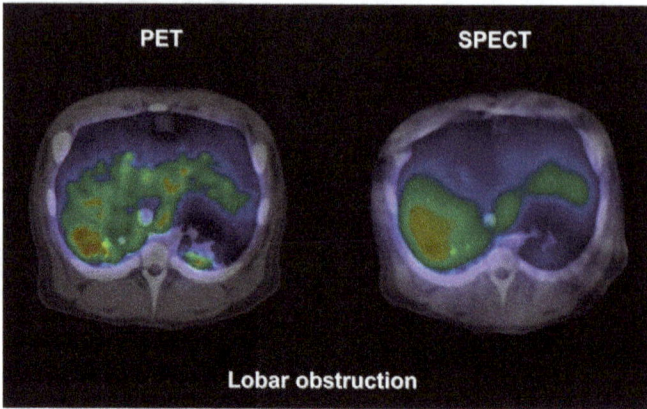

Figure 5.9:   PET/CT (^{68}Ga) and SPECT/CT (^{99m}Tc) images of lung ventilation during lower lobar obstruction. The ability of the two techniques to detect poor ventilation in the left lower lobe (lower right in the images) is similar. However, the ventilation distribution on PET image has higher spatial resolution than that on the SPECT image, perhaps suggesting diffuse bronchial constriction in other regions of the lung, which is not detected with SPECT. Both techniques provide 3D information albeit at differing spatial resolutions. Used with permission from Ref. 8.

coincidence counting serves to greatly improve the spatial resolution compared to SPECT, and this can be appreciated in Figure 5.9 where details in the PET image suggest that there are small regions of low ventilation (colored blue in the image) in the right lung that are not detectable on the lower spatial resolution SPECT image.

PET imaging is highly specialized. The tracers used generally have very short half-lives (on the order of minutes) and so must be produced close to the imaging facility, typically requiring a cyclotron to do so. Further, the radiation doses involved can be quite high and so it is often limited to clinical applications in which there is a clear benefit to obtaining the images.

5.2.4 *MRI Agents*

The use of magnetic resonance imaging (MRI) in the lung is typically quite limited due to the low density of water in the lung (typical proton MRI derives its signal from the water molecules present) and because the structure of the lung causes what little MRI signal is present to decay

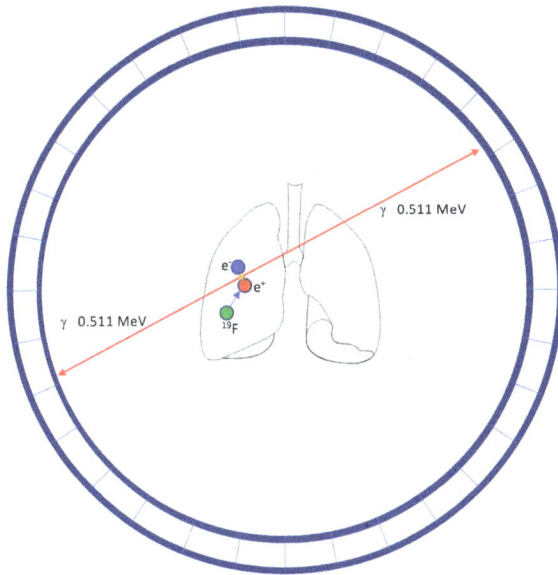

Figure 5.10: The principle of PET. A tracer labeled with a positron-emitting atom (^{19}F in this case) is used. The tracer emits a positron that immediately upon encountering an electron is annihilated, ejecting 2 gamma photons, each of 0.511 MeV energy, in opposite directions. The annihilation is known to have occurred along the line connecting the two detectors that register the photons using coincidence counting. This serves to localize the site more accurately than SPECT, improving spatial resolution.

rapidly. In order to use MRI to detect particles that have deposited in the lung, those particles need to alter the MR signal present. Broadly speaking, there are approaches to use both positive contrast (increasing the MR signal) and negative contrast (decreasing the MR signal).

Positive contrast agents for MRI are typically based around the use of gadolinium (Gd), which serves to lengthen the T1 decay time of the MR signal. Without delving into the details, MRI involves two decay times of the signal, termed T1 and T2, and by appropriate manipulation of the MR pulse sequence used in the imaging protocol, changes in one or both of these can be utilized to provide specific information. The inhaled Gd agents have been used to a very limited extent in animal models. Aerosolized Gd-DTPA, an MR contrast agent, has been used to measure ventilation in pigs and other agents have also been tested.[9] However, it is at present unclear whether this is safe for use in humans and much further development is required.

Negative contrast agents have also been utilized in animal studies. These agents are typically based on the inclusion of iron (Fe), which because of its ferromagnetic properties destroys the MR signal. The intrinsic problem with a negative contrast agent in the lung is that the MR signal ordinarily present is very low and so further destroying the signal leads to difficulties in signal-to-noise ratio of the measurement. Superparamagnetic iron oxide particles (termed MION) are used as a contrast agent (more typically as an injected contrast agent). Aerosolized iron containing particles were used to study the pattern of aerosol deposition in rat lungs[10,11] and were able to quantify deposition and examine the ratio of central to peripheral deposition. However, while the deposition occurred *in vivo*, the imaging itself was only able to be performed in the lungs after they were excised, fixed, and then imaged after being filled with fluid.

At present, the use of MRI for aerosol studies is in its infancy. Whether it will ever grow to become a useful *in vivo* tool in humans remains to be seen.

5.2.5 *Light-Based Fluorescent Imaging*

Recently, improvements in the use of direct optical imaging involving fluorescent tracers have been applied to small animal studies. Such a technique requires a sensitive light collection system and an optical pathway through the tissue surrounding the area of interest (in this case, the lungs) that is sufficiently short that some light can escape. Thus, such approaches are limited to small animals such as mice.

Despite these limitations, optical methods provide a potentially useful approach to the study of live animals as they allow repeat imaging of fluorescent tracers that have in some manner been introduced into the lung. The method uses either illumination of the intact animal from above and imaging of the light from the fluorescent tracer from above, or illumination from below with imaging from above. The devices include narrow band filters for both the illuminating light source and the fluorescent signal providing a considerable degree of specificity and limiting the background effects associated with auto-fluorescent of the tissue itself. To date, there have been few studies that have used particles in the lung[12] and it is at present unclear whether sufficient signal can be obtained from aerosolized particles deposited in the lung, but the theoretical attraction of the imaging modality is clear.

Of course, there is a significant scattering of the fluorescent light generated by the tracers in use as it passes through the tissue between its point of generation and exiting the animal's body. This serves to limit the spatial resolution of the technique, but there still remains a good degree of localization possible.[13]

5.3 Computational Models of Aerosol Deposition

As discussed in Section 5.1 of this chapter, several experimental techniques can be used to measure total and/or regional deposition of inhaled aerosols. However, the spatial resolution of deposition measurements is generally limited to a small number of regions, in particular, in human studies that mainly rely on indirect measurements. Mathematical models have often been used to complement experimental studies under different exposure conditions. These models not only help interpret experimental data but also allow predictions to be made for cases where experimental data are not available or are not ethically obtainable. Due to the complexities of the respiratory system, most early computational models of aerosol transport and deposition used a simplified representation of airway anatomy while more recent approaches have taken advantage of the developments in automated reconstruction of lung airways from MR or CT images to create highly realistic lung models in which aerosol transport and deposition can be predicted.

5.3.1 *Discrete Models of Aerosol Deposition*

5.3.1.1 *Early models*

The early models of the respiratory tract consisted of a discrete number of morphometric regions in which deposition by inertial impaction, gravitational sedimentation, and Brownian diffusion was predicted. Findensein[14] was the first to develop a model made of nine distinct morphometric regions starting with the trachea and ending with alveolar sacs. Deposition was computed by means of probabilities that a particle entering a compartment was deposited. Particles that did not deposit remained airborne and were transported to the next compartment. Deposition probabilities were estimated for each compartment k for both inspiration (d_{ki}) and expiration (d_{ke}). Total deposition (DE_{tot}) was then calculated as the sum of deposition in each compartment (DE_k):

$$DE_{tot} = \sum_{k=1}^{n} DE_k \left(d_{ki}, d_{ke} \right) \qquad (5.5)$$

Findensein calculated total deposition for particles ranging from 0.03 to 30 μm and predicted that minimum deposition occurred for particles with a diameter of ~0.2 μm. This model was later modified to include the upper airway (mouth and pharynx)[15] and to account for mixing due to pulmonary flow.[16] Such mixing often denoted as convective mixing refers to all mechanisms except for Brownian diffusion that transfer particles from the inspired air into the resident air. More detailed morphometric models were later developed: Beeckmans[17] used the symmetric model of Weibel made of 23 generations of airways[18] (Figure 2.3) while Yeh and Schum[19] developed a model that included separate airway trees for each lobe of the lung in which both total and lobar deposition could be predicted.

5.3.1.2 *The ICRP lung model*

Driven by the need to define exposure limits to airborne radionuclides in workers, the International Commission on Radiological Protection (ICRP) developed several models for deposition and retention of inhaled radioactive particles. The first model published in 1960 had a very simple structure in which the respiratory tract was divided into an upper respiratory tract (URT), and a lower respiratory tract (LRT), with no specific anatomical regions assigned to the URT and LRT.[20] The model did not take into account the effect of particle size or breathing patterns on aerosol deposition. Rather, it was assumed that 50% of an inhaled aerosol was deposited in the URT tract, 25% was exhaled, and 25% was retained in the lungs.

A more detailed model based on the work of Findensein, Landhal, and Beeckmans for deposition calculations was published in 1979.[21] The respiratory tract was described by three compartments: the naso- and oropharynx, the tracheobronchial region (trachea to terminal bronchioles), and the pulmonary region that included the respiratory bronchioles, alveolar ducts, and alveolar sacs. The third and the most advanced ICRP model published in 1994[22] includes five regions: 1) the anterior nasal passages (extrathoracic or ET1); 2) the posterior nasal passages, larynx, pharynx, and mouth (ET2); 3) the trachea and bronchi (bronchial region, BB); 4) the bronchioles (bronchiolar region, bb); and 5) the alveolar region. This latest model was refined based on numerous experimental data sets of aerosol deposition obtained in human subjects and in lung casts that were used to derive empirical deposition efficiencies. The model also takes into account the polydispersity of the aerosol and its inhalability, i.e. its ability to enter the nose and mouth during breathing. Finally, its applicability

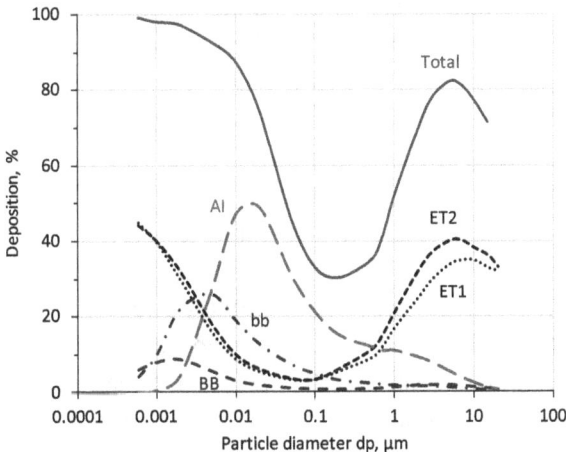

Figure 5.11. Regional and total deposition in the lung of reference workers (male Caucasian) as predicted by the 1994 ICRP model.[22] See text for the definition of the different lung regions. The total deposition is the sum of deposition in the five regions of the model.

was extended to various populations and breathing conditions. Figure 5.11 shows the effect of particle size on deposition in the five regions of the model for a reference worker (male Caucasian adult) as predicted by the ICRP model.

5.3.1.3 *Multiple path particle deposition (MPPD) models*

The discrete models described above use a single "typical" path representing the whole lung or an individual lobe in which deposition is computed. Deposition in each airway of the single path is then multiplied by the number of airways in each generation to provide an estimate of total deposition. Such an approach implies that deposition in each airway of a given generation is similar and does not account for any inhomogeneity in the branching pattern and/or subtended volume. These inhomogeneities affect flow rate in individual airways and thus also affect deposition. The development of multiple-path models has allowed this limitation to be addressed.

One of the most widely used models is the MPPD model developed by Anjilvel and Asgharian.[23] The model uses semi-empirical relationships in the URT and solves flow and deposition in the LRT made of cylindrical airways in a two-step process. First, the airflow rates and velocities in all airways of the lung are calculated, assuming that flow in an airway is proportional to the volume distal to that airway. Second, deposition is calculated using theoretically derived efficiencies for deposition by diffusion, sedimentation, and impaction within the airway or airway bifurcation. The MPPD model provides not only total deposition but also lobar-specific and airway-specific information. The model can be accessed at https://www.ara.com/products/multiple-path-particle-dosimetry-model-mppd-v-304 and can be used to assess particle deposition in rat and human lungs for a wide range of particle sizes (0.01–20 µm), breathing patterns, and functional residual capacities. Available human lung geometries include 10 distinct ages from a 3-month-old infant lung to a 21-year-old adult lung. This freely available model has been extensively validated. Lung ventilation distribution in the MPPD model has been shown to match lobar flows in healthy humans,[24,25] and predictions of particle deposition fractions have been compared favorably with measurements in rats[23] and humans.[24]

5.3.1.4 *Stochastic models*

A variant on the typical path model is a stochastic approach first proposed by Koblinger and Hofmann[26,27] that accounts for the effect of lung asymmetry. Each inspired particle moves through a single pathway selected randomly using Monte Carlo techniques from a lung model with statistically distributed airway dimensions. Deposition by impaction, sedimentation, and diffusion are computed by deterministic formulae in the intrathoracic region of the lung while upper airway deposition is based on empirical relationships.[28] Each pathway includes a number of airway bifurcation units connected in series. This approach takes into consideration the variations in diameter, length, and branching angle of airways in each generation. By simulating the random paths of many particles, typically 100,000, statistical means can be calculated for total, regional, and generational deposition. The model can also provide detailed 3D deposition patterns in the entire respiratory tract. This stochastic approach has been validated against experimental data (for example see Figure 5.12) and used in several applications such as the optimization of aerosol drug delivery[29,30] and in health risk assessment.[31]

5.3.2 *One-Dimensional (1D) Continuous Models*

Another approach to predict aerosol deposition models is based on a continuous description of aerosol transport in the lung.[34,35] This involves solving a 1D convective-diffusive equation incorporating a term accounting for deposition:

$$\frac{\partial C}{\partial t} = D\frac{s}{S}\frac{\partial^2 C}{\partial x^2} + \frac{1}{S}\frac{\partial(sD)}{\partial x}\frac{\partial C}{\partial x} - \frac{Q}{S}\frac{\partial C}{\partial x} - \frac{L}{S} \tag{5.6}$$

where C is the aerosol concentration, D is the diffusion coefficient that incorporates both Brownian diffusion and an apparent diffusion

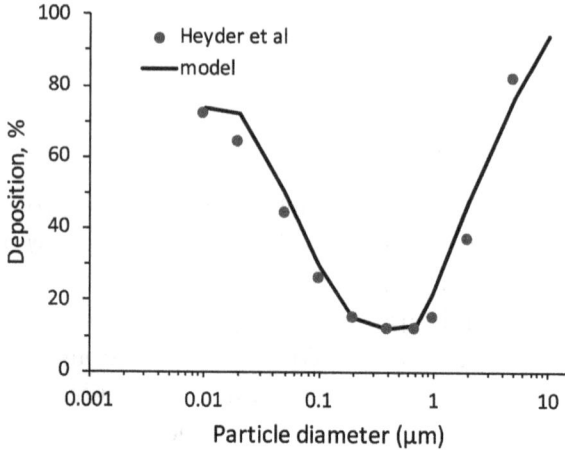

Figure 5.12. Comparison between experimental deposition values[32] and total deposition predictions from the stochastic multiple path lung model[33] for the following breathing conditions: Tidal volume = 1000 mL, breathing period = 4 s, and flow rate = 500 mL/s.

coefficient due to convective mixing, s is the airway cross-section, S is the alveoli plus airway cross-section, x is the axial coordinate (from the upper airway down to the alveolar sacs), Q is the flow rate (equal to S × mean axial velocity in airways (u)), and L is the deposition term that includes deposition by impaction, sedimentation, and diffusion (see Section 3.3).

In most studies, the lung model consists of the symmetrical model of Weibel[18] represented in the form of the so-called trumpet model where the cross section of a given generation is equal to the sum of the cross section of the individual airways belonging to that generation (Figure 2.3). While these models were originally used to predict deposition of non-hygroscopic monodisperse aerosols, later iterations have included particle hygroscopy and also particle coagulation.[36]

Unlike most of the typical path approaches that can only predict deposition for steady-state conditions with a constant flow during both inspiration and expiration, the continuous approach described here allows for predicting aerosol transport and deposition for any breathing pattern. Also, this 1D approach allows prediction of aerosol transport for any time-dependent aerosol concentration profile at the mouth. For example, Darquenne *et al.*[35,37] have used this not only to

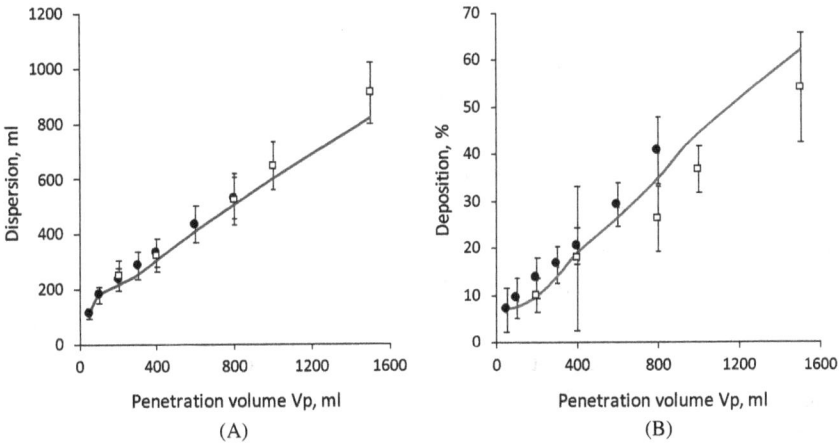

Figure 5.13. Comparison between model predictions and aerosol bolus parameters as a function of penetration volume (V_p) for 0.87-μm-diameter particles and a flow rate of 250 mL/s. (A) dispersion. (B) deposition (DE). Symbols (means ± SD) and lines refer to experimental and numerical results, respectively. Experimental data are obtained from Darquenne *et al.*[37] (□) and Brand *et al.*[38] (●); solid line: predictions from 1D model using the Weibel symmetric lung model. Modified from Ref. 37.

model total deposition from continuous aerosol inhalations but also to predict deposition (Equation 5.2) and dispersion (Equation 5.3) of aerosol boluses (Figure 5.13).

5.3.3 *Multi-Dimensional Models*

While 1D models have the advantage of being able to predict deposition throughout the entire lung, they lack the ability to describe site-specific deposition within individual airways or in specific locations in the lung. Computational fluid dynamics (CFD) models, on the other hand, use 2D or 3D geometries in which the spatial distribution of deposited particles can be predicted using detailed governing flow and particle transport equations. These models, however, are more difficult to implement, require extensive computing resources, and thus typically only focus on a specific region of the lung.

CFD models need to integrate aerosol characteristics, breathing parameters, flow patterns, and geometric features to accurately predict aerosol deposition. Most of the CFD studies assume that the aerosol is sufficiently diluted in the gas phase so that the airflow and particle transport can be computed separately. The airflow pattern is obtained by solving the Navier–Stokes equations, a set of equations that describe the transport of incompressible flows. Early studies focused on lung regions of predominantly laminar flow, i.e. medium-sized and small airways, where CFD can be used without the added complications of turbulence models.[39–41]

The numerical solution of the Navier–Stokes equations for turbulent flow is complex and, compared to laminar flows, requires a much finer mesh resolution such that the computational time becomes largely unrealistic for direct numerical simulation (DNS) in complex airway geometries. In practice, when modeling turbulent flows, time-averaged equations such as the Reynolds-averaged Navier–Stokes equations (RANS), are often used in combination with turbulence models, as this approach does not call for the same stringent mesh requirements as in the DNS method. Common turbulence models used in computing lung flows include the k–ε, k–ω, and shear-stress transport models where k is the turbulent kinetic energy, ε is its dissipation rate, and $\omega = k/\varepsilon$. Large eddy simulation (LES) can also be used to solve these equations. While the LES approach is computationally more expensive than RANS both in terms of computation time and memory, it typically produces more accurate predictions.[42,43]

One important aspect of CFD modeling is the selection of boundary conditions. For models of the upper airway, boundary conditions are fairly straightforward as there is only one outlet, although inlet conditions can get complex when simulating drug delivery from an aerosol device such as a dry powder inhaler or metered-dose inhaler. When the model includes several generations of airways and thus many outlets, the choice of boundary conditions becomes more challenging. One of the easiest choices is to assume a uniform pressure on all outlets; however, such a choice often provides erroneous flow distribution within the model. A better option is to consider a weighted outflow boundary condition where the fraction of airflow at each outlet is proportional to the volume of the distal lung beyond the outlet. This option leads to more accurate flow predictions at least in healthy lungs but requires anatomical information for distal lung volumes. Another more recent option is to couple each outlet of the 3D CFD model with 1D or 0D models that incorporate distal lung mechanics properties (see Section 5.3.4).

As mentioned above, when the aerosol is sufficiently diluted, particle transport and deposition in the CFD models can be computed separately from the flow. Particle transport is most commonly predicted through a Lagrangian approach (i.e. where each particle is tracked individually) solving Newton's second law of motion. Particle motion in the carrier gas is affected by various forces. A typical equation of motion can be expressed as

$$m_p \frac{d\vec{u}_p}{dt} = \vec{F}_D + m_p \vec{g} + \vec{F}_{Br} \tag{5.7}$$

where m_p and $\vec{u}_p$ are the particle mass and velocity respectively, $\vec{F}_D$ is the drag force, $\vec{g}$ is the gravitational acceleration, and $\vec{F}_{BR}$ is the force due to Brownian diffusion. Additional forces such as electrostatic or thermophoretic forces and near-wall turbulence effects can also be considered.

For submicron particles and/or when the particle concentration is high, the Eulerian approach is usually preferred. Unlike in the Lagrangian approach where particle transport is tracked for each particle individually, the Euler approach considers particle concentration in the transport equation that can be expressed as[44]

$$\frac{\partial \rho C}{\partial t} + \nabla.(\rho u C) = \nabla.(\Gamma \nabla C) + S_c \tag{5.8}$$

where t is the time, C is the particle concentration, ρ and v are the air density and velocity, respectively, Γ is the effective particle diffusivity (i.e. Brownian diffusivity and eddy diffusivity from turbulent flows) and S_c is a sink term accounting for particle deposition.

Equation (5.8) can be modified to account for inertia and sedimentation effects for micron-sized particles. It can also be modified to account for hygroscopy, vapor condensation, or evaporation on the particles and coagulation. Details can be found in review articles by Rostami[44] and Kleinstreuer *et al.*[45]

Several CFD studies have focused on the extrathoracic upper airway and large conducting airways, which exhibit complex geometries and turbulent/transitional flow regimes. While earlier studies were based on idealized shapes,[46–51] more recent studies have developed models derived from imaging data from individual subjects.[52–54] These models extend from the oral and/or nasal cavities down through several generations of lung airways, the number of generations often being limited by the resolution of the imaging technique. Typically, these CFD models include airways with diameter down to approximately 1–2 mm. An example is shown in Figure 5.14.

The first detailed computations of intra-acinar aerosol transport were performed using rigid models ranging from an infinitely long central channel surrounded by alveoli with circular shapes[55,56] to 2D and 3D geometries made of several generations of alveolated ducts.[57–60] Even though these CFD studies did not consider the rhythmical

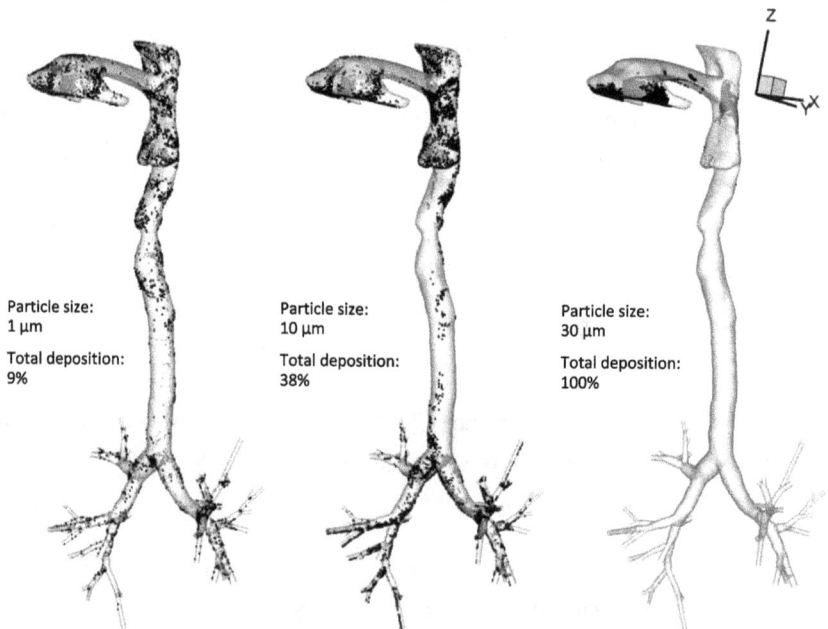

Figure 5.14. CFD-predicted deposition in a model of the upper airway and large conducting airways of a healthy male adult for three particle sizes (1, 10, and 30 μm) at a steady flow rate of 15 L/min. From Ma and Lutchen.[53]

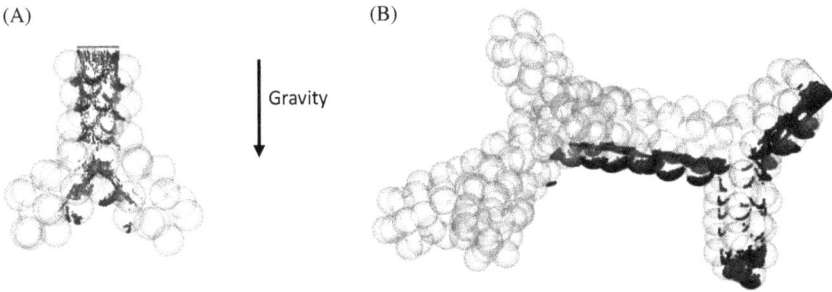

Figure 5.15. CFD predictions of alveolar deposition after a single breath (2 s inspiration, 2 s expiration). (A) Deposition of 1 µm-diameter particles in a symmetric bifurcation of alveolated ducts for a tidal volume of 0.5 L. (B) Deposition of 3 µm-diameter particles in an asymmetric 5-generation acinar model for a tidal volume of 0.9 L. Modified from Ma and Darquenne.[62]

expansion and contraction of the alveolar spaces that accompany each breath, they showed that the streamline pattern of the flow was very sensitive to alveolar duct geometry, in particular, the geometry near the alveolar aperture. They also showed that the presence of the alveolar septa contributed to the penetration of particles in the very periphery of the lung and that there were large inhomogeneities in deposition patterns within the acinar structure. Subsequent studies[61–63] have included the motion of the alveolar cavities during breathing and have highlighted the importance of convective exchange between the lumen and surrounding alveolar cavities, which significantly increase the number of particles depositing in the alveoli. An example is shown in Figure 5.15.

5.3.4 *Hybrid Models*

Despite the substantial development in computing hardware and modeling techniques, CFD studies typically only include a subregion of the respiratory system because of the prohibitive computational costs compared to lower-dimensional models. Accordingly, multiscale strategies have been developed to link different models that apply to different regions of the lung so that a realistic subject-specific picture of the fate of inhaled aerosol in the lungs can be obtained.

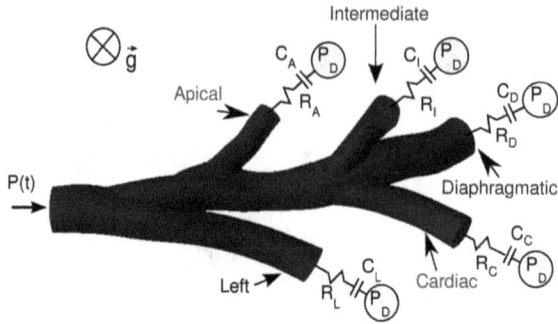

Figure 5.16. Example of a 3D rat CFD airway geometry coupled to a 0D model of the peripheral lung. From Oakes *et al.*[64] The central airways are highly realistic but the lung periphery is represented by relatively simple 0D models that are much easier to implement computationally.

One strategy has been to integrate distal lung mechanics through coupling of the 3D CFD model of the upper airway and large conducting airways with 0D or 1D models at each outlet. 0D models are represented by sets of simple ordinary differential equations representing the compliant mechanics of the airways (Figure 5.16); 1D models can be represented by trumpet models or by multi-branch-point models. While these models are still in their infancy, promising preliminary results suggest that hybrid models can accurately predict site- and region-specific deposition of aerosol throughout the respiratory system. Such models can thus be an effective tool to explore and understand the connection between disease, diagnosis, and inhaled therapy outcome.

References

1. Darquenne C, Paiva M, West JB, and Prisk GK. (1997). Effect of microgravity and hypergravity on deposition of 0.5- to 3-μm-diameter aerosol in the human lung. *J. Appl. Physiol.* **83**: 2029–2036.
2. Darquenne C, West JB, and Prisk GK. (1998). Deposition and dispersion of 1 μm aerosol boluses in the human lung: Effect of micro- and hypergravity. *J. Appl. Physiol.* **85**: 1252–1259.
3. Darquenne C, West JB, and Prisk GK. (1999). Dispersion of 0.5–2 μm aerosol in micro- and hypergravity as a probe of convective inhomogeneity in the human lung. *J. Appl. Physiol.* **86**: 1402–1409.

4. Mills CN, Darquenne C, and Prisk GK. (2002). Mode shift of an inhaled aerosol bolus is correlated with flow sequencing in the human lung. *J. Appl. Physiol.* **92**: 1232–1238.

5. Devadason SG, Chan HK, Haeussermann S, Kietzig C, Kuehl PJ, Newman S, Sommerer K, and Taylor G. (2012). Validation of radio-labeling of drug formulations for aerosol deposition assessment of orally inhaled products. *J. Aerosol Med. Pulm. Drug Deliv.* **25 Suppl 1**: S6–S9.

6. Garrard CS, Gerrity TR, Schreiner JF, and Yeates DB. (1981). The characterization of radioaerosol deposition in the healthy lung by histogram distribution analysis. *Chest* **80**: 840–842.

7. Darquenne C, Zeman KL, Sa RC, Cooper TK, Fine JM, Bennett WD, and Prisk GK. (2013). Removal of sedimentation decreases relative deposition of coarse particles in the lung periphery. *J. Appl. Physiol.* **115**: 546–555.

8. Borges JB, Velikyan I, Langstrom B, Sorensen J, Ulin J, Maripuu E, Sandstrom M, Widstrom C, and Hedenstierna G. (2011). Ventilation distribution studies comparing Technegas and "Gallgas" using 68GaCl3 as the label. *J. Nucl. Med.* **52**: 206–209.

9. Haage P, Karaagac S, Adam G, Glowinski A, and Gunther RW. (2001). Comparison of aerosolized gadoteridol and gadopentetate dimeglumine for magnetic resonance ventilation imaging of the lung. *Magn. Reson. Med.* **46**: 803–806.

10. Oakes JM, Scadeng M, Breen EC, Prisk GK, and Darquenne C. (2013). Regional distribution of aerosol deposition in rat lungs using magnetic resonance imaging. *Ann. Biomed. Eng.* **41**: 967–978.

11. Darquenne C, Borja MG, Oakes JM, Breen EC, Olfert IM, Scadeng M, and Prisk GK. (2014). Increase in relative deposition of fine particles in the rat lung periphery in the absence of gravity. *J. Appl. Physiol.* **117**: 880–886.

12. Deshmukh M, Kyutscher HL, Gao D, Sunil VR, Malaviya R, Vayas K, Stein S, Laskin JD, Laskin DL, and Sinko PJ . (2012). Biodistribution and renal clearance of biocompatible lung targeted poly(ethylene glycol) (PEG) nanogel aggregates. *J. Control. Release* **164**: 65–73.

13. Breen EC, Malloy JL, Tang K, Xia F, Fu Z, Hancock RE, Overhage J, Wagner PD, and Spragg RG. (2013). Impaired pulmonary defense against Pseudomonas aeruginosa in VEGF gene inactivated mouse lung. *J. Cell. Physiol.* **228**: 371–379.

14. Findensein W. (1935). Uber das Absetzen kleiner, in der Luft suspendierter Teilchen in der mensehlichen Lunge bei der Atmung. *Pflugers Arch.* **236**: 367–379.

15. Landahl HD. (1950). On the removal of airborne droplets by the human respiratory tract: I. The lung. *Bull. Math. Biophys.* **12**: 43–56.
16. Beeckmans JM. (1965). The deposition of aerosols in the respiratory tract. I. Mathematical analysis and comparison with experimental data. *Can. J. Physiol. Pharmacol.* **43**: 157–172.
17. Beeckmans JM. (1965). Correction factor for size-selective sampling results, based on a new computed alveolar deposition curve. *Ann. Occup. Hyg.* **8**: 221–231.
18. Weibel ER. (1963). *Morphometry of the Human Lung*. New York: Academic Press.
19. Yeh HC, and Schum GM. (1980). Models of human lung airways and their application to inhaled particle deposition. *Bull. Math. Biol.* **42**: 461–480.
20. ICRP. (1960). *Report of Committee II on Permissible Dose for Internal Radiation. ICRP Publication 2.* London: Pergamon Press.
21. ICRP. (1979). Limits for intakes of radionuclides by workers. ICRP Publication 30 (Part 1). *Ann. ICRP* **2**.
22. ICRP. (1994). *Human Respiratory Tract Model for Radiological Protection. Publication 66.* New York, NY: Pergamon Press.
23. Anjilvel S, and Asgharian B. (1995). A multiple-path model of particle deposition in the rat lung. *Fundam. Appl. Toxicol.* **28**: 41–50.
24. Asgharian B, Price OT, and Hofmann W. (2006). Prediction of particle deposition in the human lung using realistic models of lung ventilation. *J. Aerosol Sci.* **37**: 1209–1221.
25. Chang YH. (1999). A Model of ventilation distribution in the human lung. *Aerosol Sci.Technol.* **30**: 309–319.
26. Koblinger L, and Hofmann W. (1990). Monte Carlo modeling of aerosol deposition in human lungs. Part I: Simulation of particle transport in a stochastic lung structure. *J. Aerosol Sci.* **21**: 661–674.
27. Hofmann W, and Koblinger L. (1990). Monte Carlo modeling of aerosol deposition in human lungs Part II. Deposition fractions and their sensitivity to parameter variations. *J. Aerosol Sci.* **21**: 675–688.
28. Stahlhofen W, Rudolf G, and James AC. (1989). Intercomparison of experimental regional aerosol deposition data. *J. Aerosol Med.* **2**: 285–308.
29. Farkas A, Jokay A, Furi P, Balashazy I, Muller V, Odler B, and Horvath A. (2015). Computer modelling as a tool in characterization and optimization of aerosol drug delivery. *Aerosol Air Qual. Res.* **15**: 2466–2474.
30. Jvatal A, Farkas A, Balashazy I, Szabo-Revesz P, and Ambrus R. (2017). Aerodynamic properties and in silico deposition of meloxicam potassium

incorporated in a carrier-free DPI pulmonary system. *Int. J. Pharm.* **520**: 70–78.

31. Salma I, Furi P, Nemeth Z, Balashazy I, Hofmann W, and Farkas A. (2015). Lung burden and deposition distribution of inhaled atmospheric urban ultrafine particles as the first step in their health risk assessment. *Atmos. Environ.* **104**: 39–49.

32. Heyder J, Gebhart J, Rudolf G, Schiller CF, and Stahlhofen W. (1986). Deposition of particles in the human respiratory tract in the size range 0.005–15 μm. *J. Aerosol Sci.* **17**: 811–825.

33. Hofmann W, and Koblinger L. (1992). Monte Carlo modeling of aerosol deposition in human lungs. Part III: Comparison with experimental data. *J. Aerosol Sci.* **23**: 51–63.

34. Taulbee DB, and Yu CP. (1975). A theory of aerosol deposition in human respiratory tract. *J. Appl. Physiol.* **38**: 77–85.

35. Darquenne C, and Paiva M. (1994). One-dimensional simulation of aerosol transport and deposition in the human lung. *J. Appl. Physiol.* **77**: 2889–2898.

36. Robinson RJ, and Yu CP. (2001). Deposition of cigarette smoke particles in the human respiratory tract. *Aerosol Sci.Technol.* **34**: 202–215.

37. Darquenne C, Brand P, Heyder J, and Paiva M. (1997). Aerosol dispersion in human lung: Comparison between numerical simulations and experiments for bolus tests. *J. Appl. Physiol.* **83**: 966–974.

38. Brand P, Rieger C, Schulz H, Beinert T, and Heyder J. (1997). Aerosol bolus dispersion in healthy subjects. *Eur. Respir. J.* **10**: 460–467.

39. Balashazy I, and Hofmann W. (1993). Particle deposition in airway bifurcations: I. Inspiratory flow. *J. Aerosol Sci.* **24**: 745–772.

40. Zhang L, Asgharian B, and Anjilvel S. (1997). Inertial deposition of particles in the human upper airway bifurcations. *Aerosol Sci.Technol.* **26**: 97–110.

41. Asgharian B, and Anjilvel S. (1994). Inertial and gravitational deposition of particles in a square cross section bifurcating airway. *Aerosol Sci. Technol.* **20**: 177–193.

42. Liu Y, Matida EA, Gu J, and Johnson MR. (2007). Numerical simulation of aerosol deposition in a 3-D human nasal cavity using RANS, RANS/EIM, and LES. *J. Aerosol Sci.* **38**: 683–700.

43. Matida EA, Finlay WH, Breuer M, and Lange CF. (2006). Improving prediction of aerosol deposition in an idealized mouth using large-eddy simulation. *J. Aerosol Med.* **19**: 290–300.

44. Rostami AA. (2009). Computational modeling of aerosol deposition in respiratory tract: A review. *Inhal. Toxicol.* **21**: 262–290.
45. Kleinstreuer C, Zhang Z, and Donohue JF. (2008). Targeted drug-aerosol delivery in the human respiratory system. *Annu. Rev. Biomed. Eng.* **10**: 195–220.
46. Kleinstreuer C, and Zhang Z. (2003). Laminar-to-turbulent fluid-particle flows in a human airway model. *Int. J. Multiphase Flow* **29**: 271–289.
47. Stapelton KW, Guentsch E, Hoskinson MK, and Finlay WH. (2000). On the suitability of the κ-ε turbulence modeling for aerosol deposition in the mouth and throat: A comparison with experiment. *J. Aerosol Sci.* **31**: 739–749.
48. Zhang Z, Kleinstreuer C, and Kim CS. (2001). Flow structure and particle transport in a triple bifurcation airway model. *J. Fluids Eng.* **123**: 320–330.
49. Zhang Y, Finlay WH, and Matida EA. (2004). Particle deposition measurements and numerical simulation in a highly idealized mouth–throat. *J. Aerosol Sci.* **35**: 789–803.
50. Xi J, Longest PW, and Martonen TB. (2008). Effects of the laryngeal jet on nano- and microparticle transport and deposition in an approxiamte model of the upper tracheobronchial airways. *J. Appl. Physiol.* **104**: 1761–1777.
51. Gemci T, Ponyavin V, Chen Y, Chen H, and Collins R. (2008). Computational model of airflow in upper 17 generations of human respiratory tract. *J. Biomech.* **41**: 2047–2054.
52. Corley RA, Kabilan S, Kuprat AP, Carson JP, Minard KR, Jacob RE, Timchalk C, Glenny RW, Pipavath S, Cox T, Wallis CD, Larson RF, Fanucchi MV, Postlethwait EM, and Einstein DR. (2012). Comparative computational modeling of airflows and vapor dosimetry in the respiratory tracts of rat, monkey, and human. *Toxicol. Sci.* **128**: 500–516.
53. Ma B, and Lutchen KR. (2009). CFD simulation of aerosol deposition in an anatomically based human large-medium airway model. *Ann. Biomed. Eng.* **37**: 271–285.
54. Jayaraju ST, Brouns M, Lacor C, Belkassem B, and Verbanck S. (2008). Large eddy and detached eddy simulations of fluid flow and particle deposition in a human mouth–throat. *J. Aerosol Sci.* **39**: 862–875.
55. Tsuda A, Butler JP, and Fredberg JJ. (1994). Effects of alveolated duct structure on aerosol deposition in the pulmonary acinus. Part I: Diffusion in the absence of gravity. *J. Appl. Physiol.* **76**: 2497–2509.

56. Tsuda A, Butler JP, and Fredberg JJ. (1994). Effects of alveolated duct structure on aerosol deposition in the pulmonary acinus. Part II: Gravitational sedimentation and inertial impaction in the absence of diffusion. *J. Appl. Physiol.* **76**: 2510–2516.

57. Darquenne C. (2001). A realistic two-dimensional model of aerosol transport and deposition in the alveolar zone of the human lung. *J. Aerosol Sci.* **32**: 1161–1174.

58. Darquenne C. (2002). Heterogeneity of aerosol deposition in a two-dimensional model of human alveolated ducts. *J. Aerosol Sci.* **33**: 1261–1278.

59. Harrington L, Prisk GK, and Darquenne C. (2006). Importance of the bifurcation zone and branch orientation in simulated aerosol deposition in the alveolar zone of the human lung. *J. Aerosol Sci.* **37**: 37–62.

60. Sznitman J, Helmsch T, Wildhaber JH, Tsuda A, and Rosgen T. (2009). Respiratory flow phenomena and gravitational deposition in a three-dimensional space-filling model of the pulmonary acinar tree. *J. Biomech. Eng.* **131**: 131010.

61. Darquenne C, Harrington L, and Prisk GK. (2009). Alveolar duct expansion greatly enhances aerosol deposition: A three-dimensional CFD study. *Phil. Trans. Royal Soc. A Math. Phys. Eng. Sci.* **367**: 2333–2346.

62. Ma B, and Darquenne C. (2011). Aerosol deposition characteristics in distal acinar airways under cyclic breathing conditions. *J. Appl. Physiol.* **110**: 1271–1282.

63. Hofemeier P, and Sznitman J. (2016). The role of anisotropic expansion for pulmonary acinar aerosol deposition. *J. Biomech.* **49**: 3543–3548.

64. Oakes JM, Marsden A, Grandmont C, Shadden SC, Darquenne C, and Vignon-Clementel IE. (2014). Airflow and particle deposition simulations in health and emphysema: from in-vivo to in-silico animal experiments. *Ann. Biomed. Eng.* **42**: 899–914.

Chapter 6
Clearance of Particles

6.1 Introduction

As discussed in Chapter 3, there are many parameters that affect the extent and site of particle deposition within the lung. In a similar fashion, once deposited, particles are cleared by the lungs by different mechanisms depending on their deposition site (Figure 6.1). Particles that deposit in the alveolar region can be cleared by mechanisms such as phagocytosis by alveolar macrophages, particle dissolution, or movement of free particles and particle-containing cells directly into the interstitium or the lymphatics. Particles that deposit in the conducting airways are mainly removed by mucociliary clearance (MCC) and to a lesser extent by airway macrophages. Cough is also an important clearance mechanism that prevents pulmonary aspiration, promotes ciliary activity and clears airway debris. However, cough is most effective only for the upper generations of airways. The combination of mucociliary and cough clearance constitutes "mucus clearance."

The rate of the various clearance mechanisms differs by several orders of magnitude, with mucus clearance being very much the faster process (half-life of hours/day vs. months/years for alveolar clearance). Thus, small changes in aerosol deposition location have the potential to result in substantial differences in retention periods of inhaled aerosols in the respiratory tract, which in turn may significantly affect the level of toxicity from particulate matter.

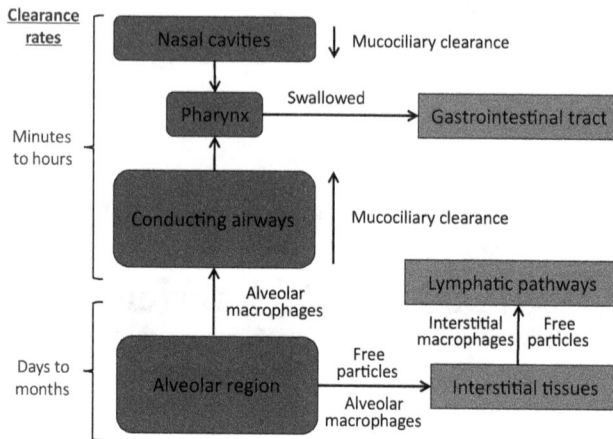

Figure 6.1: Schematic representation of the major clearance mechanisms of insoluble particles in the lung

6.2 Mucociliary Clearance

Mucociliary clearance is the primary clearance mechanism of foreign pathogens and inhaled particles from the conducting airways and nasal mucosa. Airway surfaces are lined with ciliated epithelial cells and covered with an airway surface layer (ASL) made of two main components: a mucus or gel layer that entraps foreign pathogens and inhaled particles and a low-viscosity periciliary layer (PCL) that provides cell-surface lubrication and enables ciliary beating for efficient mucus transport (Figure 2.9).

6.2.1 *Cilia*

There are about 10^9 cilia per cm^2 of airway surface with cilia being longer and more densely packed in the large airways than in the bronchioles (Figure 2.8). In the trachea, cilia are about 6 μm long and have a diameter of ~250 nm; in the intermediate airways, they are about 3–4 μm long with a diameter of 100 nm. In healthy lungs, cilia beat in a coordinated, directional wave-like pattern, referred to as metachronal waves, at a frequency estimated to be ~10–20 Hz[1] (Figure 6.2). The mucus and entrapped particles are constantly transported towards the pharynx to be swallowed or expectorated.

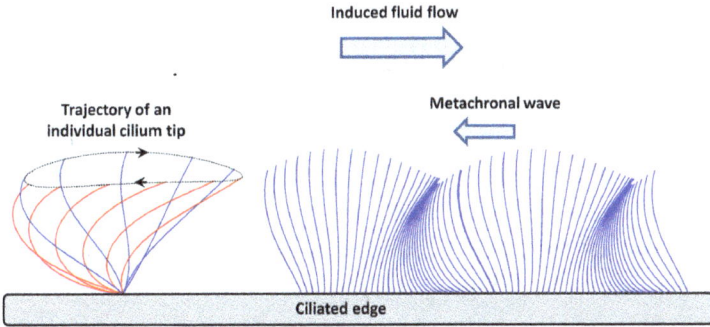

Figure 6.2: Schematic representation of the stroke of an individual cilium and of a group of cilia to induce motion by metachronal waves. See text for details. From Ref. 2.

6.2.2 *Airway Surface Layer*

The ASL is made of a mucus layer overlying a PCL that is in contact with the epithelial cells on the airway surface. Along with the ciliated epithelial cells, the airway surface is lined with mucus-secreting goblet cells and other secretory cells. The goblet cells are mainly located in the trachea and large airways and become less frequent in the bronchioles. Airway mucus is also produced by submucosal glands that are only found in cartilaginous airways. These submucosal glands are the major source of airway mucus and consist of mucous and serous cells lining a common secretory duct leading to the airway epithelial surface. Both the quantity and composition of the secretions are affected by the autonomic nervous system and can be altered by mechanical or chemical irritation.

In healthy lungs, mucus contains 97% water and 3% solids and forms a viscoelastic gel. Most of the solids are mucin glycoproteins (~30%) with the remaining constituents being non-mucin proteins, lipids, salts, and cellular debris.[3] The height of the mucous layer varies throughout the airway tree and is about 2–5 µm thick in the trachea. It should be noted that the mucus layer covers only part of the tracheobronchial tree, with discrete mucous plaques in the smaller airways and a consolidated mucous sheet in the large airways.

The PCL is composed of a low-viscosity liquid that provides an efficient medium for ciliary beating. It also serves as a barrier to prevent foreign pathogens and particles from reaching the cell surface. Traditionally thought to be mainly composed of water, it has recently been proposed that the PCL also contains large amounts of mucins and large glycoproteins that are tethered to the cilia to create a fine mesh that prevents larger molecules such as inhaled particles to penetrate the PCL.[4] In normal airways, the PCL approximates the length of the extended cilia (approximately 7 μm) to ensure efficient mucociliary transport (Figure 2.9).

6.2.3 *Mucociliary Clearance*

The rate of MCC is not only dependent on the rate of ciliary beating but also strongly influenced by the hydration state of the ASL. Thus, control of the water balance in the airways is essential. Water is secreted by serous cells in the surface epithelium and in the submucosal glands by active chloride secretion. Water can also be secreted by plasma transudation, a mechanism that becomes an important contributor following local irritation or widespread pulmonary inflammation. Water is removed by active sodium transport across the surface epithelium. In airway diseases, the balance is shifted from water secretion to mucus secretion. This results in a highly concentrated (i.e., more viscous) ASL that is poorly moved by the cilia and results in accumulation of secretions in the airways. In bronchitis and asthma, this is mainly due to conversion of serous glands to mucous cells. In cystic fibrosis, serous gland cells cannot secrete water because they lack functioning chloride channels in their membrane due to an impaired cystic fibrosis transmembrane conductance regulator protein.

Mucus velocity values are the highest in the trachea and decrease with increasing airway generation. In healthy humans, velocities have been reported in the range of 5.5–14 mm/min in the trachea, 1–2.4 mm/min in the upper bronchial airways and 0.4–0.6 mm/min in the lower bronchial airways.[5,6] Combined with water absorption along the tracheobronchial tree, the difference in mucus velocities between the peripheral and proximal airways ensure that secretions do not accumulate in the central airways.

The time frame for MCC is on the order of hours. Clearance from the ciliated nasopharyngeal region is completed within about 4 h, and clearance from the ciliated epithelium of the tracheobronchial tree is completed within 24 h.

6.3 Macrophages

The main clearance mechanism for insoluble particles depositing in the alveolar region is the uptake by alveolar macrophages or phagocytosis. Alveolar macrophages are large mononuclear cells comprising 95% of the free cells in the alveolar region. The rate of phagocytosis depends on particle size, surface composition and density. Typically, the larger the particle size, the slower the phagocytosis. However, there is also evidence that very small particles in the nanometer range clear at a slower rate than micron-size particles.[7] Most of the macrophages with engulfed particles migrate towards the terminal bronchioles and are cleared through the mucociliary system. However, because the alveolar macrophages live only for weeks and the migration of these macrophages towards the mucociliary escalator is a slow process, the engulfed particles may be released when the macrophages die and be taken up by other alveolar macrophages. Even though this process may result in some of the particles persisting in the lung indefinitely, most of the particle-laden macrophages are cleared within weeks to months. It has also been suggested that macrophages with phagocytized particles migrate across the epithelium into the interstitium and then into the thoracic lymph nodes (see Section 6.4). However, this process only affects a very small fraction of particle-carrying alveolar macrophages and is not a major clearance mechanism.[8]

In the early 1990s, new evidence suggested that particles that deposited in the conducting airways could also be phagocytized by airway macrophages. Gehr and colleagues[9] showed that a considerable number of particles, initially deposited in the conducting airways, could be found closely associated with the airway epithelium and that the presence of an airway surfactant film at the mucus-air surface might facilitate the penetration of deposited particles into the mucus towards the epithelium by interfacial forces. Airway macrophages may then phagocytize those particles and lead to long-term retention in this region. Uptake into airway epithelial cells has also been described.[10]

6.4 Translocation to the Interstitium, Lymphatic System and/or Blood

A fraction of insoluble particles that deposit in the alveoli are translocated into the pulmonary interstitium. Most of these are free particles as opposed to particles engulfed in alveolar macrophages. Particles reach the interstitial space by endocytosis and subsequent exocytosis mainly by type I epithelium cells. These particles can then bound to connective tissue and stay in the interstitium indefinitely, or they can be transported into the lymphatics or, less frequently, enter the blood circulation. As mentioned above, most of the particles that deposit in the alveolar region of the lung are cleared by alveolar macrophages and only a very small fraction of them are transported to the interstitium. However, when the pulmonary particle burden is excessively high, a situation referred to as overload conditions, alveolar macrophage-mediated clearance is inhibited and the translocation of particles from the alveoli into the lung's interstitial spaces is increased. Particle size and surface characteristics also affect particle penetration into the interstitium with smaller particles being translocated to a greater extent than particles in the micron size range.

Particles that penetrate the interstitium can migrate through the lymphatic drainage system. The pulmonary lymphatic system is a network of vessels connecting aggregates of lymphoid tissue that drains excess fluid, proteins, cells and particles from the pulmonary interstitium. In the lumen of the lymphatic vessels, funnel-shaped, one-way valves work with vascular and pulmonary pressures to maintain a steady unidirectional flow of lymph from the lung periphery to the larger lymphatic collecting vessels. These vessels feed through highly organized lymphatic tissue that finally reach the hilar and tracheo-bronchial lymph nodes before the fluid in them enters the blood stream. Particle clearance through the lymphatic system is a very slow process with particle migration taking months to years to complete.

6.5 Absorption of Soluble Particles

In addition to MCC, soluble particles depositing in the conducting airways are removed by absorptive mechanisms. The apical membranes of the cells lining the airway lumen, i.e., the membranes in contact with the PCL, are joined by tight junctions that control the passage of ions and neutral species through the intercellular space. Hydrophilic molecules can either pass through these tight junctions or be actively transported intracellularly via endocytosis and exocytosis. Non-polar molecules with high lipid and low water solubility (lipophilic molecules) pass easily through the cell membrane by passive diffusion. From the submucosal region, particles are then absorbed into either the systemic circulation, the bronchial circulation or the lymphatic system. The same mechanisms of absorption apply to soluble particles depositing in the alveolar region of the lung. Absorption of substances through the alveolar epithelium into the blood circulation and/or lymphatic system is however faster than absorption through the airways epithelium.

While clearance by mucociliary transport and by macrophage phagocytosis are defense mechanisms that have evolved to protect the lungs from exposure to foreign particulates, they are also barriers to inhaled drug delivery and present a challenge for the development of therapeutic aerosols. Although macromolecules can be absorbed into the systemic circulation over several hours, they can be rapidly taken up by alveolar macrophages and/or removed by mucociliary transport. On the other hand, small solutes delivered to the lungs quickly diffuse across lung epithelia and penetrate the bloodstream within minutes.

6.6 Particle Translocation Beyond the Lungs

Inhaled particles that deposited in the lung can be found in small but measurable quantities in other organs. In most cases, the presumed pathway is the bloodstream following gradual solution in lung fluids and diffusion into pulmonary capillaries.[11] In a rat exposure study using ultrafine particles (<100 nm), while particles deposited in both the conducting airways and lung periphery were predominantly cleared via airways and larynx into the gastrointestinal tract and feces, a small fraction of ultrafine particles were translocated to secondary target organs (liver, spleen, heart, brain, <1%) and carcass (<5%) 7 days after inhalation.[12] The translocation of ultrafine particles was dependent on particle size with the translocation fraction of 15 nm particles being one order of magnitude larger than that of 80 nm particles. Extrapulmonary particle uptake over a six-month period decreased with time in liver, spleen, heart and brain when compared to data obtained during the first 7 days after inhalation.[13] Ultrafine carbon particles (20–29 nm) were also found to be effectively translocated to the liver in rats 1 day after exposure.[14] Data obtained in animals should however be applied with caution to humans. Indeed, a study in humans showed no significant translocation of inhaled 35 and 100-nm carbonaceous particles to the systemic circulation (<1%) and extrapulmonary organs over a 24-h period.[15,16]

Besides extrapulmonary translocation of ultrafine particles via the blood circulation, neuronal pathways from deposits on the nasal olfactory mucosa to the brain via the olfactory nerve have been identified. Early studies in squirrel monkeys showed the translocation of intranasally instilled 50-nm colloidal gold particles to the olfactory bulbs via olfactory nerves.[17] A later study found significant and continuous increases of 36-nm carbonaceous particles in the olfactory bulb of rats throughout a 7-day period after aerosol exposure and provided strong arguments favoring axonal transport of the ultrafine particles via olfactory neurons from nasal deposits into the central nervous system as the major translocation mechanism.[13] This direct path for ultrafine particles into the central nervous system, bypassing the tight blood-brain barrier, could present potential risks of neurotoxic effects. However, considering that only 5% of the human nasal mucosa is olfactory epithelium as opposed to 50% in rodents,[18] one can question the importance of olfactory nerve translocation for ultrafine particles in humans.

6.7 Measurement of Particle Clearance

Gamma scintigraphy (see Section 5.2.1) is the most commonly used imaging technique to measure *in vivo* MCC function. An aerosol of radiolabeled (typically ^{99m}Tc) particles is inhaled, while the total radio-activity in the lung is measured over time by a gamma camera, typically up to 24 h post-aerosol exposure. MCC rates can then be measured by assuming that the radiolabeled particles that deposited on the air-way surface move out of the lung at the same rate as the airway secretions in which they are immersed. These measures essentially aim at assessing how effective the mucociliary system is at clearing mucus and associated bacteria, deposited particulate matter and/or toxins from the lungs. This is of particular importance in airway diseases such as asthma, chronic bronchitis and cystic fibrosis (Figure 6.3) where MCC can be substantially impaired, leaving patients prone to exacer-bation of airway inflammation resulting from the accumulation of bacteria and toxins on airway surfaces. Controlled inhalation of the radiolabeled aerosols is also important for optimizing intrasubject repeatability of MCC measures.

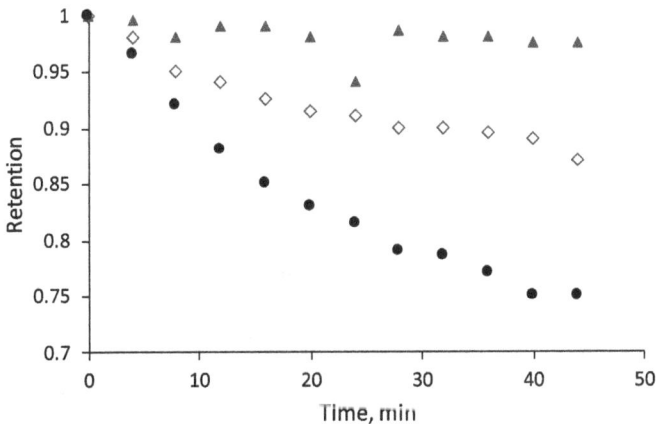

Figure 6.3: Averaged retention of radiolabeled particles that deposited in the right lung as a function of time post-inhalation in healthy subjects (•, $N = 12$), mild-to-moderate (◊, $N = 20$) and severe (▲, $N = 5$) cystic fibrosis patients. Retention is cal-culated as decay-corrected activity measured at the different time points normalized by activity measured immediately post-aerosol inhalation. Data are obtained from Ref. 19.

Alveolar clearance can be assessed by measuring activity counts over a period of several days or weeks until the activity of the radiolabeled particles has decayed to a point where reliable measurements can no longer be made. Long-term clearance kinetics can also be studied by a technique called magnetopneumography following the inhalation of magnetic iron oxide particles.[20] The advantage of the magnetic labeling technique compared with radioactive labeling is that it has no physical decay constant, and thus, it allows for measurements to be made for periods of up to 1 year.

Retention curves can be characterized by two phases. The first one is fast with clearance half-times between 6 and 12 h (Figure 6.4A). It is completed by convention within 24 hours and represents MCC of particles from the conducting airways. The second phase is much slower with a half-time of weeks or even months (Figure 6.4B) and represents particle clearance from the alveolar region by macrophage activity and/or dissolution.

Particle clearance rates are highly dependent on regional deposition in the lung. Particles depositing in the proximal airways clear at a faster rate than those depositing in the small airways. It is thus

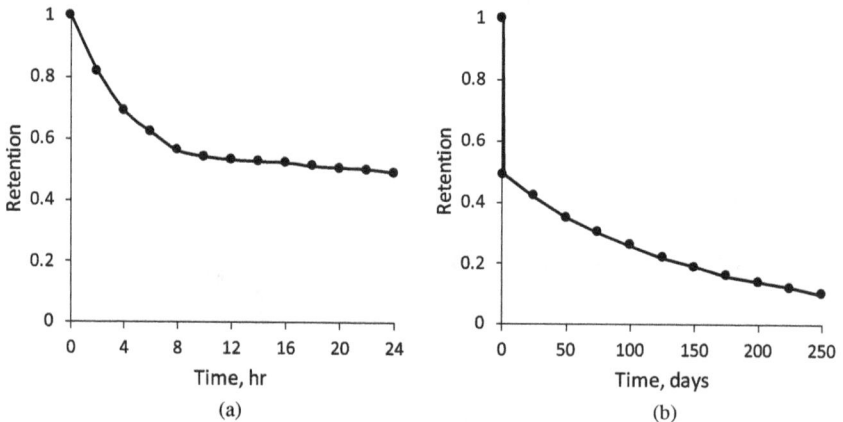

Figure 6.4: Retention of 2 µm-diameter ferromagnetic iron oxide particles deposited in the lungs of 13 healthy non-smokers. Data show mean values. (A) Retention during the first 24 h following inhalation. (B) Retention within 250 days post-inhalation. Modified from Ref. 20.

important to characterize the initial regional deposition. One of the most commonly used indices is the ratio of deposited particles in the central and peripheral region of the lung, i.e., the C/P ratio. These regions of the lung are defined on a gas equilibrium or transmission scan as illustrated in Figure 5.7A and are displayed over the aerosol scans to determine the initial counts in each region (Figure 5.7B). To account for the difference in relative lung volume between the two regions, the ratio of central to peripheral activity counts is normalized by the C/P ratio for the gas equilibrium or transmission scan, where the resulting C/P ratio provides an index of relative deposition between the two regions. Because the central region outlines both bronchial airways and lung parenchyma around them, a C/P of ≈1 reflects primarily homogenous deposition throughout the pulmonary airspaces. Increases in C/P to values >1 reflect an increase in central vs. peripheral deposition mainly through increased bronchial deposition.

Activity measurements at 24 h post-inhalation, i.e., the 24-h retention (R_{24}), primarily represent the fraction of aerosol initially deposited in the non-ciliated or alveolar region. Conversely, the 24-h clearance (i.e., $1-R_{24}$) reflects the deposition in the entire tracheo-bronchial tree that could be cleared by ciliary action.[22] Intermediate time points between initial retention and R_{24} reflect deposition from proximal to distal airways as retention times progress. To assess tracheobronchial retention (TB R_t) over time, i.e., clearance kinetics from only the MCC-dependent airways, R_{24} is subtracted from the intermediate retention measurements and normalized by deposition in the tracheobronchial tree, i.e.,

$$TB\ R_t = (R_t - R_{24})/(1 - R_{24}) \tag{6.7.1}$$

where $t < 24$ h.

Gamma scintigraphy is useful not only to determine dysfunctional mucociliary apparatus in subjects with airway disease but also to measure the efficacy of drugs designed to improve clearance of airway secretions. For example, this technique has been used to demonstrate that the inhalation of hypertonic saline significantly improves the clearance of secretions in cystic fibrosis patients.[23]

References

1. Livraghi A, and Randell SH. (2007). Cystic fibrosis and other respiratory diseases of impaired mucus clearance. *Toxicol. Pathol.* **35**: 116–129.
2. Bottier M, Peña Fernández M, Pelle G, Isabey D, Louis B, Grotberg JB, and Filoche M. (2017). A new index for characterizing micro-bead motion in a flow induced by ciliary beating: Part II, modeling. *PLoS Comput. Biol.* **13**: e1005552.
3. Munkholm M, and Mortensen J. (2014). Mucociliary clearance: Pathophysiological aspects. *Clin. Physiol. Funct. Imaging* **34**: 171–177.
4. Button B, Cai L-H, Ehre C, Kesimer K, Hill DB, Sheehan JK, Boucher RC, and Rubinstein M. (2012). A periciliary brush promotes the lung health by separating the mucus layer from airway epithelia. *Science* **337**: 937–941.
5. Foster WM, Langenback E, and Bergofsky EH. (1980). Measurement of tracheal and bronchial mucus velocities in man: Relation to lung clearance. *J. Appl. Physiol.* **48**: 965–971.
6. Morrow PE, Gibb FR, and Gazioglu KM. (1967). A study of particulate clearance from the human lungs. *Am. Rev. Respir. Dis.* **96**: 1209–1221.
7. Oberdorster G. (2001). Pulmonary effects of ultrafine particles. *Int. Arch. Occup. Environ. Health* **74**: 1–8.
8. Oberdorster G. (1993). Lung dosimetry: Pulmonary clearance of inhaled particles. *Aerosol. Sci. Technol.* **18**: 279–289.
9. Gehr P, Schurch S, Berthiaume Y, Im Hof V, and Geiser M. (1990). Particle retention in airways by surfactant. *J. Aerosol. Med.* **3**: 27–43.
10. Sorokin SP, and Brain JD. (1975). Pathways of clearance in mouse lungs exposed to iron oxide aerosols. *Anat. Rec.* **181**: 581–625.
11. Lippmann M, Yeates DB, and Albert RE. (1980). Deposition, retention, and clearance of inhaled particles. *Br. J. Ind. Med.* **37**: 337–362.
12. Kreyling WG, Semmler M, Erbe F, Mayer P, Takenada S, Schulz H, Oberdorster G, and Ziesenis A. (2002). Translocation of ultrafine insoluble iridium particles from lung epithelium to extrapulmonary organs is size dependent but very low. *J. Toxicol. Environ. Health A* **65**: 1513–1530.
13. Oberdorster G, Sharp Z, Atudorei V, Elder A, Gelein R, Kreyling W, and Cox C. (2004). Translocation of inhaled ultrafine particles to the brain. *Inhal. Toxicol.* **16**: 437–445.

14. Oberdorster G, Sharp Z, Atudorei V, Elder A, Gelein R, Lunts A, Kreyling W, and Cox C. (2002). Extrapulmonary translocation of ultra-fine carbon particles following whole-body inhalation exposure of rats. *J. Toxicol. Environ. Health A.* **65**: 1531–1543.

15. Wiebert P, Sanchez-Crespo A, Falk R, Philipson K, Lundin A, Larsson S, Moller W, Kreyling WG, and Svartengren M. (2006). No significant translocation of inhaled 35-nm carbon particles to the circulation in humans. *Inhal. Toxicol.* **18**: 741–747.

16. Wiebert P, Sanchez-Crespo A, Seitz J, Falk R, Philipson K, Kreyling WG, Moller W, Sommerer K, Larsson S, and Svartengren M. (2006). Negligible clearance of ultrafine particles retained in healthy and affected human lungs. *Eur. Respir. J.* **28**: 286–290.

17. De Lorenzo AJD. (1970). The olfactory neuron and the blood–brain barrier. In: *Taste and Smell in Vertebrates*, edited by Wolstenholme GEW, and Knight J. London: J.&A. Churchill, pp. 151–176.

18. Harkema JR. (1992). Epithelial cells of the nasal passages. In: *Comparative Biology of the Normal Lung*, edited by Parent RA. Boca Raton, FL: CRC press, pp. 27–36.

19. Regnis JA, Robinson M, Bailey DL, Cook P, Hooper P, Chan H-K, Gonda I, Bautovich G, and Bye PTP. (1994). Mucociliary clearance in patients with Cystic Fibrosis and in normal subjects. *Am. J. Respir. Crit. Care. Med.* **150**: 66–71.

20. Moller W, Haussinger K, Winkler-Heil R, Stahlhofen W, Meyer T, Hofmann W, and Heyder J. (2004). Mucociliary and long-term particle clearance in the airways of healthy nonsmoker subjects. *J. Appl. Physiol.* **97**: 2200–2206.

21. Darquenne C, Zeman KL, Sa RC, Cooper TK, Fine JM, Bennett WD, and Prisk GK. (2013). Removal of sedimentation decreases relative deposition of coarse particles in the lung periphery. *J. Appl. Physiol.* **115**: 546–555.

22. Bennett WD, Herbst M, Alexis NE, Zeman KL, Wu J, Hernandez ML, and Peden DB. (2011). Effect of inhaled dust mite allergen on regional particle deposition and mucociliary clearance in allergic asthmatics. *Clin. Exp. Allergy.* **41**: 1719–1728.

23. Donaldson SH, Bennett WD, Zeman KL, Knowles MR, Tarran R, and Boucher RC. (2006). Mucus clearance and lung function in cystic fibrosis with hypertonic saline. *N. Engl. J. Med.* **354**: 241–250.

Chapter 7
Aerosols as a Diagnostic Tool

7.1 Introduction

As discussed in Chapter 5 (Section 1.2), aerosol bolus inhalations have been extensively used to study deposition in specific volumetric regions of the lung. Aerosol bolus inhalations may also be used as a physiological test to measure convective mixing, ventilation distribution and/or airspace size.

7.2 Aerosol Bolus Dispersion

7.2.1 *Convective Mixing and Ventilation Heterogeneity*

Convective mixing refers to all the transport mechanisms except Brownian diffusion that irreversibly transfer inspired air into resident air and can be studied using aerosol bolus inhalations. A particle with minimal intrinsic mobility acts as a non-diffusing gas closely following the air streamlines and thus can be used to study pulmonary mixing that does not result from molecular diffusion. Intrinsic mobility results from particle inertia, sedimentation and diffusion. None of these intrinsic properties are effective for particle transport in the size range 0.5–0.8 μm, particle size typically used to study convective mixing.

Aerosol bolus tests consist of inserting a small amount of aerosol (a bolus) at a predetermined point in the subject's inspiratory volume and analyzing the distribution of the aerosol bolus in the subsequent exhalation (see Chapter 5). During the inspiratory phase, the bolus divides into several segments that become more numerous as the bolus penetrates deeper into the lung. The segments recombine during expiration in such a way that the expired bolus is spread over a larger volume than the inspired bolus, indicating that particles are irreversibly transferred from the bolus to the adjacent air during a breath (Figure 5.4).

Figure 7.1A illustrates the increased spreading of exhaled boluses with increasing penetration volumes (V_p) following the inhalation of a 0.87 μm-diameter aerosol bolus with a half-width of 20 mL. Mechanisms of particle movements that contribute to convective mixing include non-reversibility of velocity profiles within the airspaces, airway and alveolar geometries, asymmetries between inspiratory and expiratory flows, cardiogenic mixing, and heterogeneous ventilation of the lung.[1] Interestingly, the linearity of the increase in bolus dispersion with increasing penetration volume (Figure 7.1B) strongly suggests that convective mixing processes in the periphery of the lung have mixing coefficients that are similar to those representative of

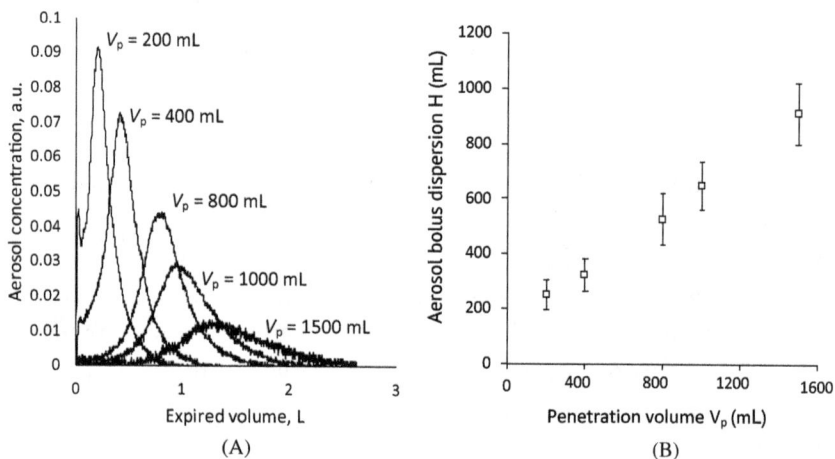

Figure 7.1: (A) Experimental tracings of 0.87-μm-diameter particles for various penetration volumes (V_p) obtained in one healthy subject at a flow rate of 250 mL/s. (B) Aerosol bolus dispersion (H) as a function of V_p averaged over ten subjects (mean ± SD) for 0.87 μm-diameter particles and a flow rate of 250 mL/s. Modified from Ref. 2.

mixing in the central airways. However, given the difference in geometry and in flow patterns between the central airways and the acinus, acinar mixing likely results from different mechanisms than those occurring in the central airways.

Ventilation heterogeneity is one of the most significant contributors to convective mixing. This has been confirmed by experiments performed in altered gravitational environments[3] (see Chapter 11). Indeed, ventilation inhomogeneities are highly sensitive to gravity. Because the lung distorts under its own weight, the alveoli at the base of the lung are relatively compressed compared with the apical alveoli and because poorly expanded alveoli are more compliant, ventilation is higher near the bottom of the lung and becomes progressively lower near the top. Changes in gravity level, and thus in lung weight, affect the distribution of ventilation and as a consequence convective mixing. It should however be noted that any inhomogeneity in the topographical distribution of ventilation per se will not result in any increase in convective mixing without the presence of asynchronous filling and emptying of lung regions.

The effect of gravity on convective mixing is shown in Figure 7.2 as the slope of the linear regression between dispersion and

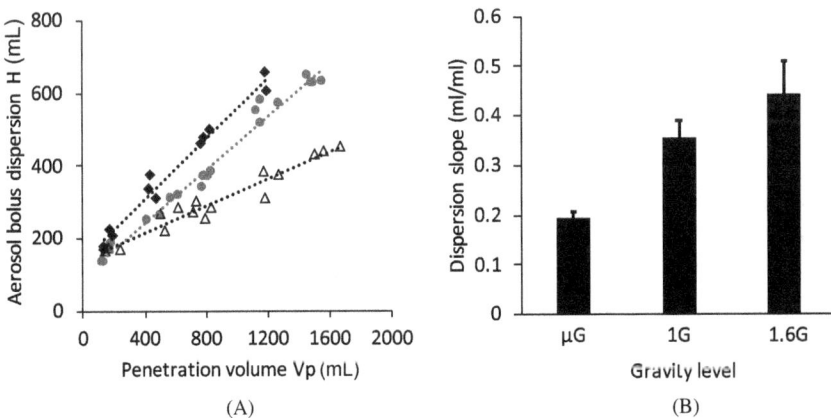

Figure 7.2: (A) Aerosol bolus dispersion as a function of penetration volume obtained in one healthy subject in μG (open triangles), 1G (closed circles) and 1.6G (closed diamonds) for 0.5 μm-diameter particles. (B) Slope of the regression lines of aerosol bolus dispersion as a function of penetration volume averaged over four healthy subjects. Data from Ref. 3.

penetration volume (V_p-H slope) in microgravity (μG), normal gravity (1G) and hypergravity (~1.6G) for 0.5 μm-diameter particles. The V_p–H slope in microgravity is at least half of that in normal gravity, suggesting that non-gravitational convective ventilatory inhomogeneities are at least as large as gravitational convective ventilatory inhomogeneities, a result consistent with studies of gas mixing.[4] The slope in μG also demonstrates the presence of significant gravity-independent convective ventilatory inhomogeneity. Such direct observation of convective inhomogeneity in the acinar region of the lung cannot be made when using gases because convective effects cannot be separated from the diffusive effects that dominate gas transport in the acinus.[1]

7.2.2 Effect of Disease on Aerosol Bolus Dispersion

Aerosol bolus dispersion not only has the sensitivity to detect changes in ventilation distribution induced by changes in gravity levels in healthy subjects, but more importantly, it can also detect alterations in airway flow patterns and ventilation distribution resulting from lung disease. For example, compared to healthy subjects, aerosol bolus dispersion is increased in patients with asthma,[5] cystic fibrosis,[6] mild-to-moderate chronic obstructive pulmonary disease (COPD)[7] and emphysema.[8] Increased dispersion has also been measured in smokers.[9,10] Increased dispersion is likely the result of regional variations in airway resistance and in the compliance of subtended acinar units that together create heterogeneities in regional time constants. The different time constants result in asynchrony of regional ventilation, which leads to an increase in the width of the expired bolus. While aerosol bolus dispersion measurements have not been shown to provide significant additional information to traditional lung function tests such as FEV_1 in subjects with moderate-to-severe disease, it may play an important role in the early detection of lung impairment in asymptomatic subjects. For example, aerosol dispersion has been shown to be significantly increased in smokers with normal lung function (as evidenced by spirometry) when compared to lifelong non-smokers.[10]

7.3 Aerosol-Based Measurement of Airspace Dimensions

There are two main aerosol-based approaches used to estimate airspace dimensions *in vivo*. The first one, referred to as the aerosol-derived airway morphometry (ADAM) technique, provides information on the airway dimensions by comparing inhaled and exhaled concentrations of monodisperse micron-sized aerosol particles. The technique uses particles in the range of 0.8–1.2 μm taking advantage of the constant settling velocity of these particles in still air, which is achieved during breath-holding. The second technique referred to as airspace dimension assessment (AiDA) uses nanoparticles (<0.1 μm) for which Brownian diffusion is the dominant transport mechanism during breath-holding from which airspace dimensions are estimated.

7.3.1 *Aerosol-Derived Airway Morphometry*

The ADAM technique is based on a series of inhalations of a monodisperse micron-sized aerosol followed by a breath-hold during which particles settle by gravity at a constant velocity; some of them depositing on airway and acinar walls. The smaller the airspace, the faster the particles are removed from the air and the fewer are recovered in the exhaled air. These aerosol inhalations are repeated for different breath-hold times with particle concentrations being measured at the mouth during both the inhalation and the exhalation following the breath-hold. Flow rates are controlled and kept below ~0.4 L/s to avoid significant deposition by inertial impaction during inhalation. Particle loss is determined as the difference between the number of inhaled and exhaled particles. The rate of particle loss as a function of breath-hold times is then used to derive effective airway diameters (EADs).

There are three versions of the ADAM technique, each providing increasing degrees of anatomical resolution. The first one is the single-breath recovery technique that consists of a full inhalation of aerosols followed by a breath-hold and an expiration. For each breath-hold, the total recovery of particles R is measured as

$$R = \frac{N_{ex}}{N_{in}} \tag{7.1}$$

where N_{in} and N_{ex} are the number of inhaled and exhaled particles, respectively. Using a model based on a system of randomly oriented tubes, EAD can be computed in terms of the half-life $t_{1/2}$, which is the breath-hold time required for one-half the particles to deposit.[11,12] The half-life $t_{1/2}$ is typically obtained on a plot of $ln\,R$ versus breath-hold time t with values for $t_{1/2}$ ranging between 20 and 30 s in healthy subjects.[12] EAD is then expressed as

$$EAD = \frac{4}{\pi\,ln\,2}\,v_s t_{1/2} \tag{7.2}$$

where v_s is the particle settling velocity. This approach provides a single value of EAD that is the volume-weighted mean EAD for the entire lung.

In contrast to the single breath recovery approach, the bolus recovery technique offers higher resolution of regional lung dimensions by computing EADs at multiple preselected lung depths. This technique uses a narrow aerosol bolus inhaled to a specific penetration volume so that only a small volumetric fraction of the lung is probed at a time. Particle recovery is then plotted as a function of breath-hold time and EAD computed using Eq. (7.2). By delivering boluses to different depths (i.e., different values of V_p), EAD values can be determined for as much of the lung as desired.

Finally, the particle concentration technique is similar to the single-breath recovery technique in that it uses whole breaths of aerosols but differs in the analysis of the exhaled air. Aerosol concentration measurements of the exhaled air are compartmentalized into increments of equal volume, each containing aerosol originating from different lung depths. The recovery from each volume increment is then based upon the change in particle concentration C within that increment and defined as

$$R = \frac{C_{ex}}{C_{in}} \quad (7.3)$$

where C_{in} and C_{ex} are the inhaled and exhaled concentrations in a given volume increment, respectively. For each increment, an EAD representative of the relatively limited mixture of airway and acinar generations containing the particles during the breath-hold can then be calculated. Because of the large number of volume increments that can be defined in a breath, this method provides more regional information about EAD than either of the other two methods.

The ADAM techniques have been shown to provide detailed information on airway diameters in healthy subjects[12–15] and also in subjects with emphysema for which EAD values are significantly higher than that for healthy controls.[16–18] Figure 7.3 summarizes

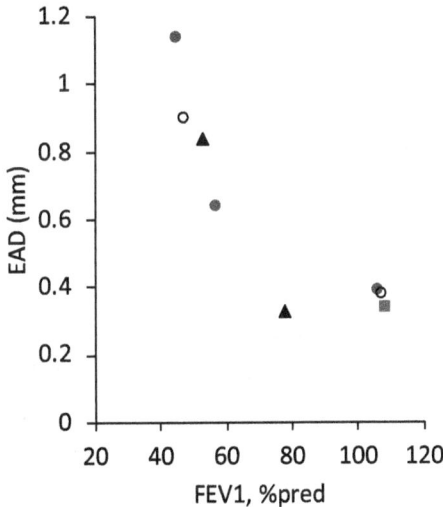

Figure 7.3: Effective airway diameter (EAD) as a function of FEV_1. EAD was obtained for a volumetric lung depth of 800 mL and is shown as average for each studied group. • Data obtained from Ref. 17 (healthy, $N = 36$; COPD [chronic bronchitis and emphysema], $N = 16$; α_1-antitrypsin (severe emphysema), $N = 9$); ▲ Data obtained from Ref. 19 (no emphysema, $N = 30$; emphysema, $N = 20$); ▪ Data obtained from Ref. 13 (healthy, $N = 79$); ○ Data obtained from Ref. 20 (healthy, $N = 11$; emphysema, $N = 24$).

average EAD values from several studies in healthy subjects and COPD patients.[13,17,19] Data are plotted as a function of FEV_1 and show a significant increase in EAD values between healthy subjects ($FEV_1 \geq 80\%$pred) and COPD patients ($FEV_1 < 80\%$pred).

7.3.2 *Airspace Dimension Assessment with Nanoparticles*

Recently, a non-invasive method to estimate distal airspace size by a series of single breath-hold nanoparticle inhalations has been proposed with the potential of circumventing difficulties in maintaining controlled and low flow rates during micron-sized aerosol inhalations as required by ADAM. Indeed, the need for a highly controlled breathing maneuver at a low flow rate in the ADAM technique makes it difficult to measure the peripheral airspace dimensions at larger volumetric lung depths and at maximum inflation. Compared to micron-sized particles, nanoparticles (<0.1 μm) have a higher ability to penetrate into the peripheral airways and are less sensitive to obstructions and disturbances to the airflow in the tracheobronchial tree. Nanoparticles with neutral electrical charge deposit almost exclusively by Brownian diffusion. Deposition by this mechanism depends on the residence time and the distance to the airspace wall, but not on the airway or alveoli orientation (see Chapter 3, Section 3.3.1.3). Similar to particle loss by gravitational sedimentation in the ADAM technique, particle loss by diffusion during a breath-hold is related to the size of the airspaces.

The breathing protocol mimics that used for measuring the diffusing capacity of the lung (DL_{CO}). The subject breathes particle-free air for a few tidal breaths, and then performs an exhalation to residual volume. This is followed by a full inhalation of nanoparticles to total lung capacity, a breath-hold of up to 20 s and an exhalation. A sample volume of ~300 mL corresponding to a volumetric lung depth of 1.2–1.5 L is collected from the exhaled air. Particle recovery is then calculated as the ratio between the aerosol concentration of the exhaled sample and the concentration of the inhaled aerosol. Recovery of nanoparticles has been shown to be independent of flow rate[21] and dependent on particle size and breath-hold times (Figure 7.4). As some diffusion also occurs during inhalation and exhalation, residence time is estimated in an analogous fashion as for the measurement of

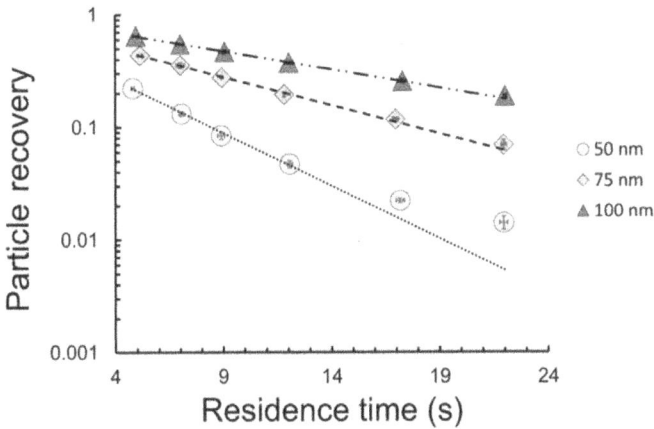

Figure 7.4: Effect of particle size and residence time on particle recovery in one healthy subject following the AiDA breathing protocol (see text for details). The lower the nanoparticles, the lower the recovery. From Ref. 21.

DL_{CO}, i.e., from 30% of the inspiratory time to the middle of the sample collection time.[22]

Similarly to the ADAM technique that produces an EAD, the AiDA technique provides a mean radius of the probed airspaces that can be expressed as

$$r = 2.89\sqrt{Dt_{1/2}} \qquad (7.4)$$

where D is the Brownian diffusion coefficient and $t_{1/2}$ is the breath-hold time required for one-half the particles to deposit.[23] Although still in its infancy, the AiDA technique has been used both in healthy subjects and in patients with COPD.[24,25] Larger values for particle recovery have been found in the COPD group than in the healthy controls, consistent with larger airspaces in the COPD group.[24]

References

1. Darquenne C, and Prisk GK. (2005). Aerosols in the study of convective acinar mixing. *Respir. Physiol. Neurobiol.* **148**: 207–216.
2. Darquenne C, Brand P, Heyder J, and Paiva M. (1997). Aerosol dispersion in human lung: comparison between numerical simulations and experiments for bolus tests. *J. Appl. Physiol.* **83**: 966–974.

3. Darquenne C, West JB, and Prisk GK. (1999). Dispersion of 0.5–2 μm aerosol in μG and hypergravity as a probe of convective inhomogeneity in the lung. *J. Appl. Physiol.* **86**: 1402–1409.
4. Verbanck S, Linnarsson D, Prisk GK, and Paiva M. (1996). Specific ventilation distribution in microgravity. *J. Appl. Physiol.* **80**: 1458–1465.
5. Schulz H, Schulz A, Brand P, Tuch T, Von Mutius E, Erdl R, Reinhardt D, and Heyder J. (1995). Aerosol bolus dispersion and effective airway diameters in mildly asthmatic children. *Eur. Respir. J.* **8**: 566–573.
6. Anderson PJ, Blanchard JD, Brain JD, Feldman HA, McNamara JJ, and Heyder J. (1989). Effect of cystic fibrosis on inhaled aerosol boluses. *Am. Rev. Respir. Dis.* **140**: 1317–1324.
7. Darquenne C, Lamm WJ, Fine JM, Corley RA, and Glenny RW. (2016). Total and regional deposition of inhaled aerosols in supine healthy subjects and subjects with mild-to-moderate COPD. *J. Aerosol Sci.* **99**: 27–39.
8. Kohlhaufl M, Brand P, Scheuch G, Meyer T, Schulz H, Haussinger K, and Heyder J. (2000). Aerosol morphometry and aerosol bolus dispersion in patients with CT-determined combined pulmonary emphysema and lung fibrosis. *J. Aerosol Med.* **13**: 117–124.
9. Anderson PJ, Hardy KG, Gann LP, Cole R, and Hiller FC. (1994). Detection of small airway dysfunction in asymptomatic smokers using aerosol bolus behavior. *Am. J. Respir. Crit. Care Med.* **150**: 995–1001.
10. Brand P, Tuch T, Manuwald O, Bischof W, Heinrich J, Wichmann HE, Beinert T, and Heyder J. (1994). Detection of early lung impairment with aerosol bolus dispersion. *Eur. Respir. J.* **7**: 1830–1838.
11. Heyder J. (1975). Gravitational deposition of aerosol particles within a system of randomly oriented tubes. *J. Aerosol Sci.* **6**: 133–137.
12. Gebhart J, Heyder J, and Stahlhofen W. (1981). Use of aerosols to estimate pulmonary air-space dimensions. *J. Appl. Physiol.* **51**: 465–476.
13. Brand P, Rieger C, Beinert T, and Heyder J. (1995). Aerosol derived airway morphometry in healthy subjects. *Eur. Respir. J.* **8**: 1639–1646.
14. Blanchard JD, Heyder J, O'Donnell CR, and Brain JD. (1991). Aerosol-derived lung morphometry: Comparisons with a lung model and lung function indexes. *J. Appl. Physiol.* **71**: 1216–1224.
15. Bennett WD, and Smaldone GC. (1987). Human variation in the peripheral air-space deposition of inhaled particles. *J. Appl. Physiol.* **62**: 1603–1610.
16. Bennett WD, and Smaldone GC. (1988). Use of aerosols to estimate mean air-space size in chronic obstructive pulmonary disease. *J. Appl. Physiol.* **64**: 1554–1560.

17. Beinert T, Brand P, Behr J, Vogelmeir C, and Heyder J. (1995). Peripheral airspace dimensions in patients with COPD. *Chest* **108**: 998–1003.

18. Brand P, Kohlhaufl M, Meyer T, Selzer T, Heyder J, and Haussinger K. (1999). Aerosol-derived airway morphometry and aerosol bolus dispersion in patients with lung fibrosis and lung emphysema. *Chest* **116**: 543–548.

19. Kohlhaufl M, Brand P, Rock C, Radons T, Scheuch G, Meyer T, Schulz H, Pfeifer KJ, Haussinger K, and Heyder J. (1999). Noninvasive diagnosis of emphysema: Aerosol morphometry and aerosol bolus dispersion in comparison to HRCT. *Am. J. Respir. Crit. Care Med.* **160**: 913–918.

20. Lehnigk B, Schleiss M, Brand P, Heyder J, Magnussen H, and Jorres RA. (2007). Aerosol-derived airway morphometry (ADAM) in patients with lung emphysema diagnosed by computed tomography — Reproducibility, diagnostic information and modelling. *Eur. J. Med. Res.* **12**: 74–83.

21. Jakobsson JKF, Hedlund J, Kumlin J, Wollmer P, and Londahl J. (2016). A new method for measuring lung deposition efficiency of airborne nanoparticles in a single breath. *Sci. Rep.* **6**: 36147.

22. MacIntyre N, Crapo RO, Viegi G, Johnson DC, van der Grinten CPM, Brusasco V, Burgos F, Casaburi R, Coates A, Enright P, Gustafsson P, Hankinson J, Jensen R, McKay R, Miller MR, Navajas D, Pedersen OF, Pellegrino R, and Wanger J. (2005). Standardisation of the single-breath determination of carbon monoxide uptake in the lung. *Eur. Respir. J.* **26**: 720–735.

23. Löndahl J, Jakobsson JKF, Broday DM, Aaltonen HL, and Wollmer P. (2017). Do nanoparticles provide a new opportunity for diagnosis of distal airspace disease? *Int. J. Nanomedicine* **12**: 41–51.

24. Aaltonen HL, Jakobsson JKF, Diaz S, Zackrisson S, Piitulainen E, Londahl J, and Wollmer P. (2018). Deposition of inhaled nanoparticles is reduced in subjects with COPD and correlates with the extent of emphysema: proof of concept for a novel diagnostic technique. *Clin. Physiol. Funct. Imaging* **38**: 1008–1014.

25. Aaltonen HL, Kindvall SS, Jakobsson JKF, Londahl J, Olsson LE, Diaz S, Zackrisson S, and Wollmer P. (2018). Airspace dimension assessment with nanoparticles reflects lung density as quantified by MRI. *Int. J. Nanomedicine* **13**: 2989–2995.

Chapter 8
Aerosol Therapeutics

The use of the inhaled route for the delivery of therapeutic compounds (drugs) has a long-established history, particularly in the case of the delivery of β2 agonists for the purposes of bronchodilation. Utilization of the inhaled route as opposed to a systemically introduced drug has potential advantages. In the case of drugs which the intended site of action is in the lung itself, there is a clear case to be made for the inhalation and deposition of the drug directly into the airways where it can act on sites such as the bronchial smooth muscle (in the case of a β2 bronchodilator) or be absorbed into the pulmonary circulation directly from the airways as might be the case with a pulmonary vasodilator.[1] Drugs delivered via the airways for systemic action may also be potentially usefully delivered through inhalation as a means to bypass the possible degradation of the drug active compound as it passes through the liver, potentially increasing their bioavailability.

There are many classes of drugs and within each class, there are many drugs, and it is not the intent of this chapter to list and describe them all. Rather, we strive to provide a broad overview of the instances in which inhaled drug therapy is useful.

8.1 Drugs Classes

8.1.1 *Bronchodilators*

To date, the most common drug delivered by inhalation is the short-acting bronchodilator, typically a β2 agonist (a short-acting beta-agonist or SABA) such as albuterol (salbutamol in Europe and some other countries). Such drugs are the mainstay of short-term asthma treatment and rescue from acute bronchoconstriction events. Non-β2 selective adrenergic agents such as epinephrine and isoproterenol have also been delivered in a similar manner, but these have fallen from favor as their non-selectivity for the β2 pathway leads to greater side effects.

Similarly, there are short-acting muscarinic agents (SAMA) also delivered by inhalation. Although these agents are generally poorly absorbed into the circulation, they can enter the airway epithelium where they act on the M1 and M3 muscarinic receptors in airway smooth muscle.

Both classes of drug (SABA and SAMA) have more recently become available in long-acting forms (LABA and LAMA) and are primarily used for maintenance therapy for asthma (LABAs) and chronic obstructive pulmonary disease (LAMAs). It is worth noting that LABAs as monotherapy for the control of asthma have been associated with an increase in asthma deaths. The increase in the number of deaths has been associated with the drug acting only to control symptoms of asthma while failing to treat the underlying inflammation associated with the disease. As a result, the use of LABAs alone for asthma control is now discouraged. Instead, they are now typically dispensed in combination with inhaled corticosteroids (ICS) that reduce inflammation in the airways.

8.1.2 *Inhaled Corticosteroids*

It is undoubtedly true that the development and deployment of ICS for the control of asthma has been a huge step forward in the treatment of the disease. All ICS are synthetic glucocorticosteroids. In addition to their intended anti-inflammatory action, they also have the effect of increasing the rate of transcription of beta-agonists,[2] making the use of combination therapy with an inhaled LABA more effective.

The use of ICS (which is usually long-term, often lifelong) causes side effects, many of which arise from oral and pharyngeal deposition that occurs during inhalation. Much of this is swallowed, providing a pathway for the systemic delivery of the ICS, and so consideration of how rapidly this is cleared by the liver (some exhibit complete first-pass metabolism, and some do not) may be an important consideration in the choice of ICS used in the long-term treatment. In addition to the systemic delivery, ICS deposition in the upper airway is associated with an increase in thrush and other fungal infections, and so rinsing of the mouth and throat following inhalation is considered good practice.

There are now triple-combination inhalers appearing on the market that contain an ICS, a LABA, and a LAMA. These are primarily aimed at the COPD patient who also has evidence of reactive airways and so can potentially benefit from all three medication classes.

8.1.3 *Inhaled Pulmonary Vasodilators*

Pulmonary vasodilators are another class of drug where aerosolized delivery is an attractive target. Pulmonary hypertension is a potentially devastating disease that is difficult to diagnose and treat. It is characterized by excessive constriction of the pulmonary vessels with the associated increase in pulmonary vascular pressures. The administration of pulmonary vasodilators has been shown to be effective. However, one of the problems associated with treatment is that pulmonary vasodilators when delivered systemically tend to cause systemic vasodilation as well, an unwanted and potentially dangerous side effect. There are multiple pathways to cause vasodilation in the pulmonary vasculature and one drug that is effective, although only in a limited number of patients, is inhaled nitric oxide (NO, a gas). Because NO is rapidly scavenged by hemoglobin, the inhaled (gas) route is effective as the NO can act on the pulmonary vasculature and be scavenged before reaching the systemic circulation. While NO is a gas, this serves to show how effective the inhaled drug delivery route can be.

Other vasodilator agents are now also available for inhalation, including Treprostinil and Iloprost, both of which are prostacyclin analogs. Both are available in inhaled formulations although the need for multiple doses per day using a nebulizer, due to the short half-life of the drugs once delivered, is still burdensome to patients.

8.1.4 *Aerosolized Antimicrobial Agents*

Inhaled antibiotics have now become or are becoming one of the mainstay therapies in chronic lung diseases such as cystic fibrosis (CF). Characterized by high viscosity mucus and resultant lung infections, the inhaled route for the delivery of antibiotics directly to infected lungs is attractive and has been shown to be somewhat effective. This began with Tobramycin but now includes several other antibiotics. The use of inhaled antibiotics is often associated with other inhaled therapies such as anti-mucolytic agents and hypertonic saline therapy. These adjunct therapies aim to break up the mucus and mucus plugging that is characteristic in CF to allow the delivery of the inhaled antibiotic to the affected areas of the lung. One of the obvious problems associated with inhaled drug delivery in cases of mucus plugging is that the inhaled agent cannot reach beyond a plugged airway, the very site where its action is most likely desired.

Other examples of antimicrobial drug delivery via inhalation include aerosolized pentamidine for the treatment of pneumocystis pneumonia and antivirals such as ribavirin and zanamivir used in the treatment of the influenza virus.

8.1.5 *Novel and Emerging Approaches for Aerosolized Therapies*

Aerosolized gene therapy, although still in its infancy, presents a number of potentially useful lung disease targets. These include CF and alpha-1 antitrypsin deficiency. The object of such therapy is to deal with the underlying genetic disorder via the delivery of functional copies of the aberrant gene. Given both diseases manifest themselves with significant problems in the lung, direct delivery to the affected organ is appealing. As repeated dosing will likely be required, there are significant issues associated with how the genes are vectored to their target (using viral or non-viral vectors). There have been numerous small clinical trials targeting CF, and while evidence of gene transfer has been seen, many have experienced problems with inflammatory responses that serve to limit efficacy.[3]

Aerosolized vaccination also represents an interesting target. As many vaccines cannot be administered via an oral route, inhalation would present a potentially convenient route of administration. This approach is even less advanced than gene therapy, but a number of pre-clinical studies have suggested that it may be feasible and effective. The best vaccine developed to date is a measles vaccine, but this is still far from ready for widespread vaccination use. However should this become effective this would serve to likely improve the ability to make measles vaccination more widespread, especially in developing countries, where the disease is widespread, and current vaccination levels are low.[3]

8.1.6 *Systemic Drug Delivery from Aerosolized Drugs*

Lung has a huge surface area and receives virtually the entire cardiac output, making it an attractive target for the delivery of drugs that cannot be delivered by an oral route and also for the administration of a drug in which a rapid action is required. While many such drugs are delivered by injection, the apparent non-invasive nature of the aerosolized route is an attractive target.

An example of the rapidity and ease of delivery via the inhaled route can be appreciated is nicotine. Although not generally used clinically except in cases of smoking cessation therapy, for which there is a nicotine inhaler available, the delivery of nicotine either by smoking or more recently by vaping is a clear example of both effective systemic drug delivery and rapid drug availability.

An attractive target for inhaled system therapy is insulin. Insulin cannot be delivered by an oral route or through transdermal patches, making injection necessary. Given the typically life-long dependence of patients on routine delivery of insulin, the need for daily (or multiple times per day) injections is unpleasant for patients and represents a significant burden to them. Early in the 2000s, an inhaled form of insulin was developed but was ultimately withdrawn after reductions in the diffusing capacity of the lungs was recognized as a side effect. More recently, a dry powder form of inhaled insulin has reached the market, utilizing pre-filled drug cartridges and a small dry powder inhaler (DPI).[4]

There are other drug formulations under development for the aerosolized delivery of systemically active drugs, but at this time it is unclear that whether inhaled drug delivery of drugs not destined for the pulmonary system will become a major component of future formularies.

8.2 Aerosol Delivery Systems

8.2.1 *Nebulizers*

Nebulizers are devices to generate aerosols from a liquid, in which the drug is dissolved or suspended. The device is designed to take the liquid and generate droplets from that liquid, which can then be inhaled. In order to do this, energy needs to be used to break the liquid into droplets. That energy source is typically what is used to define the nebulizer type: pneumatic, ultrasonic, or vibrating mesh.

8.2.1.1 *Pneumatic nebulizers*

Pneumatic nebulizers depend on a source of high-pressure air or oxygen delivered from either a compressor or a high-pressure gas source. In its simplest form, a pneumatic nebulizer consists of a capillary tube, one end of which is immersed in the liquid to be nebulized (Figure 8.1). Across the top of this is the high-pressure flow of gas, the velocity of which serves to reduce the pressure at the top of the capillary tube (Bernoulli effect). This serves to draw the liquid up the capillary tube and when it encounters the gas jet, the liquid is sheared off forming droplets. The resultant droplet cloud is propelled by the gas flow towards the outlet of the nebulizer to be inhaled. The nebulization results in a large range of particle sizes being produced, and most devices incorporate baffles or other geometric flow disruptors so that the very large droplets impact these and the liquid is returned to the nebulizer reservoir. The smaller particles however will travel with the

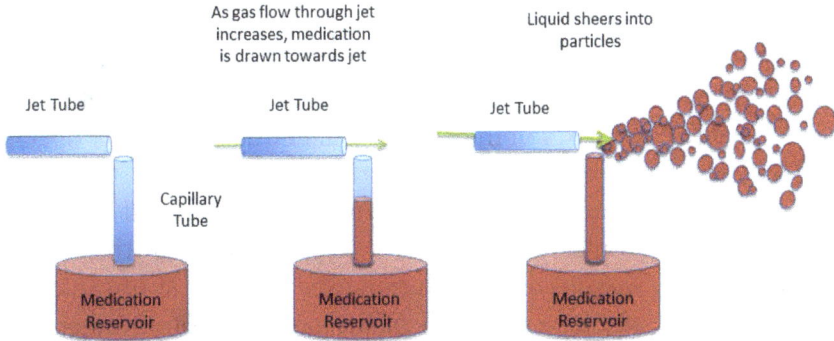

Figure 8.1: The conceptual design of a pneumatic nebulizer. The jet of air passing over the tip of the capillary tube draws liquid up the tube. As the liquid reaches the top, it is sheared off forming droplets. (Reproduced with permission from the International Society for Aerosols in Medicine [ISAM]).

airflow (just as smaller particles bypass the early stages of cascade impactors, see Chapter 4) and reach the exit of the device. A useful review of the large amount of knowledge on nebulizer design and operation can be found in the book by Finlay.[5]

In the context of delivering a drug to a patient, it is important to consider the (typically large) differences between doses at different stages of nebulization. The Nominal Dose is that placed in the nebulizer. However not all of the liquid is nebulized leading to a smaller Emitted Dose. The Inhaled Dose is smaller again, indicating that when a subject is breathing on a continuously running nebulizer, the device is emitting drug even when the subject is exhaling. Finally, the Respirable Dose is smaller again because some of the droplets generated by the device are sufficiently large that they do not reach the lungs, but instead deposit in the upper airway. A common means of attempting to characterize this is the fine-particle fraction, which is the percentage of the emitted aerosol that is smaller than 5 μm in size (or sometimes smaller than 3.5 μm). Overall, for a given nominal dose placed in a nebulizer, it is often the case that only ~10% is actually delivered to the lungs of the patient.

There are multiple types of nebulizers in use ranging from continuous output (always-on) with and without a reservoir to recapture large aerosol droplets, to nebulizers with different inspiratory and expiratory paths (potentially avoiding room contamination as excess aerosol can be collected on a filter), to breath-actuated nebulizers. Similarly, there are numerous factors that serve to affect nebulizer output: baffles, efficiency of the drug chamber design, whether operation is continuous, orientation (many are required to be vertical), gas flow and gas pressure, liquid viscosity, room humidity and temperature (affecting droplet evaporation or hygroscopic growth), liquid surface tension, suspension vs. solution, and the nature of the drug itself. Certainly, the generalization of the operation of an otherwise unspecified "generic nebulizer" is not possible.

8.2.1.2 *Ultrasonic nebulizers*

Ultrasonic nebulizers utilize high-frequency acoustic energy to generate the aerosol. Like a pneumatic nebulizer, the drug is in solution or suspension in a reservoir at the base of which is a piezoelectric crystal (Figure 8.2). This is actuated by a high-frequency electrical signal, typically in the 1.2–2.4 MHz range, and the resulting acoustic energy is delivered to the reservoir. The result is a series of standing capillary waves at the liquid surface that grow in amplitude, and droplets are generated at the crest of the wave.

The droplet size ejected from the wave is proportional to the wavelength of the standing wave, which is in turn dependent on the inverse of the driving frequency squared, inversely proportional to the density of the liquid and directly proportional to the surface tension of the liquid, all raised to the power 1/3.[6] Thus, altering the frequency of the electrical signal to the piezoelectric crystal will alter the aerosol size with a higher frequency producing smaller droplets.

As a general rule, the ultrasonic nebulizers produce a more uniform droplet size than pneumatic nebulizers, but the devices perform less well with suspensions because the particles in suspension are not necessarily well entrained into the droplets formed. Further, the acoustic energy can raise the temperature of the liquid in the reservoir quite considerably, which can be a factor with temperature-sensitive formulations. They however have the advantage of producing higher aerosol nebulization rates and higher aerosol cloud densities than pneumatic devices.

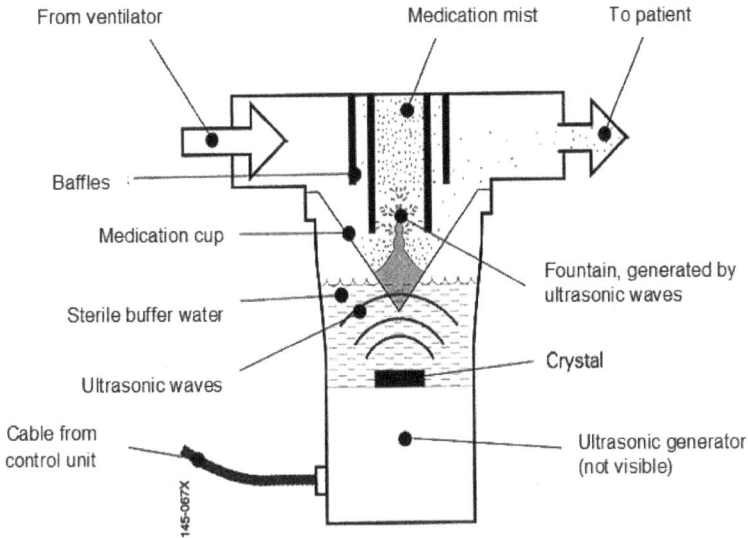

Figure 8.2: Cutaway diagram of an ultrasonic nebulizer. The ultrasonic waves generated by the piezoelectric element are passed to the medication cup, where they establish standing capillary waves. At the crest of these waves, droplets shear off and form an aerosol cloud. Larger droplets will deposit on the baffles or settle back to the medication cup for re-nebulization, while the smaller droplets are carried by the flow indicated in this figure as from the ventilator to the patient. (Reproduced with permission from the International Society for Aerosols in Medicine [ISAM]).

8.2.1.3 *Vibrating mesh nebulizers*

Vibrating mesh nebulizers also utilize ultrasonic energy to generate the aerosol, but rather than depending on standing wave generation, the liquid is forced through an aperture plate, through which a series of tiny holes have been machined. The liquid forced through the plate forms a small stream (filament) on the other side, which rapidly breaks into droplets due to the surface tension of the liquid (Figure 8.3). The surface tension of the liquid, the hole size, and the rapidity of filament formation all contribute to droplet size generated. By machining different hole sizes, droplet size can be changed, and by altering the number of holes, nebulizer output can be changed.

There are two major configurations of vibrating mesh nebulizers, passive and active. In the passive form, the aperture plate is separated from the piezoelectric drive unit by the liquid to be nebulized. In the

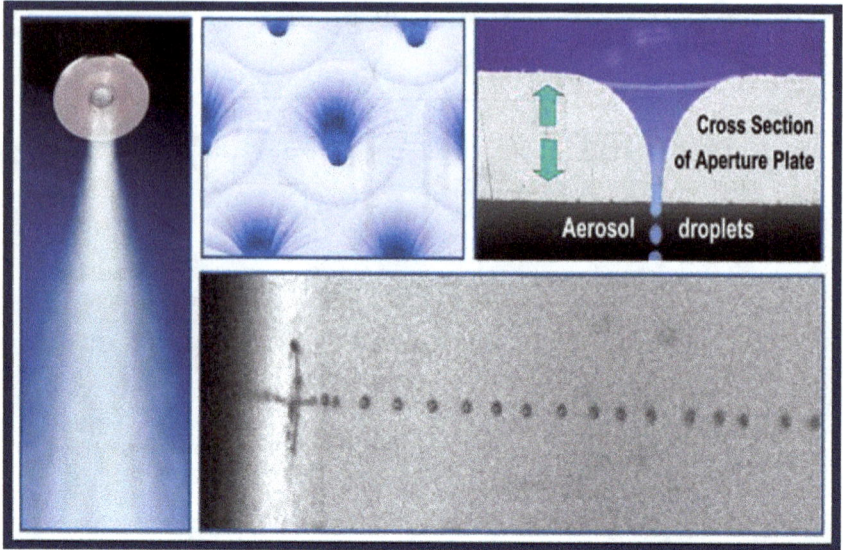

Figure 8.3: Details of a vibrating mesh nebulizer (in this example, the active form). The plate in the center of the device (left) has carefully machined holes through it, in this case, funnel-shaped apertures, as shown in the upper center and upper right. A piezoelectric crystal vibrates the plate that ~130 kHz. As the plate flexes by ~1 μm, the liquid is forced through the holes and filament of fluid formed breaks into droplets as a result of surface tension (lower right panel). (Reproduced with permission from the International Society for Aerosols in Medicine [ISAM]).

active form, the aperture plate itself is driven by the piezoelectric drive unit and the plate is moved up and down, creating an alternating pressure at the opening of the holes, forcing the liquid through.

One advantage of the active design is the ability to nebulize very small (and precise) volumes of liquid. With the device operating, a single drop can be placed on the aperture plate and it is then completely nebulized.

The other clear advantage of vibrating mesh nebulizers (both passive and active designs) is that of precise and uniform droplet size. This is a direct consequence of the precisely machined holes in the aperture plate, which serves to make for a specific droplet size (all other considerations regarding viscosity and surface tensions of the liquid being held constant).

8.2.2 *Pressurized Metered Dose Inhalers*

To date, the most common form of inhaled drug delivery in asthma, and the concept that comes to mind for most people when thinking about pharmaceutical drug inhalation is the pressured metered-dose inhaler (pMDI). These asthma "puffers" are convenient, being self-contained and small enough to fit into a pocket or purse.

Figure 8.4 shows a schematic of a typical pMDI. The drug is dissolved or suspended in the liquid, which is also the propellant, and this is contained in the cannister. Excipients or other substances such as surfactant may also be present depending on the formulation involved. Until a decade or two ago, the propellant was typically a chlorofluorocarbon (CFC) but this has subsequently been replaced with hydrofluoroalkane (HFA) as a result of concerns regarding CFC effects on the ozone layer. At the valve end of the cannister, a small

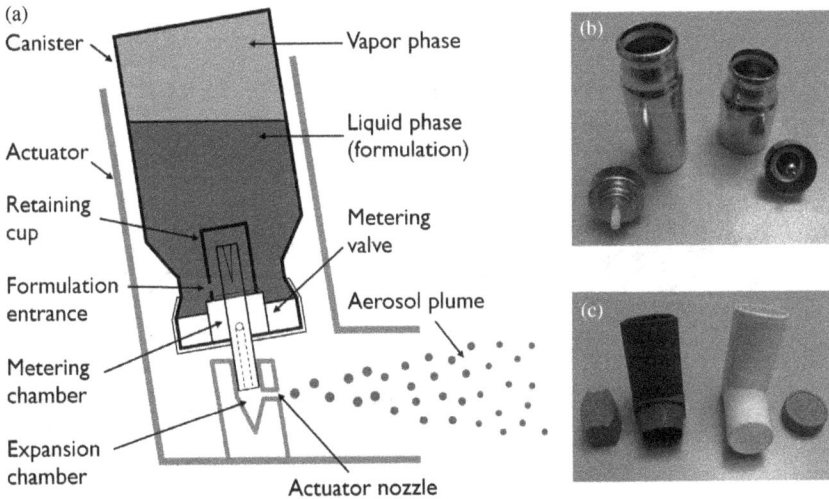

Figure 8.4: A typical pMDI configuration. Drug is either dissolved or suspended in the liquid phase of the propellant. Before actuation, the metering chamber fills with drug and when the metering valve is actuated, the contents of that chamber are ejected into the expansion chamber in the actuator body. The rapid expansion causes the propellant to boil and a cloud of aerosol particles is ejected as a plume. (Reproduced with permission from the International Society for Aerosols in Medicine [ISAM]).

metering chamber contains a valve actuated by pressing the cannister in a holder. The metering chamber fills with the drug-containing liquid and then the valve is actuated; the propellant rapidly empties the metering chamber into an expansion chamber in the holder and in doing so, aerosolizes the liquid. The effect is to dispense a preset amount of liquid (and thus a preset dose of drug) as an aerosol that can be inhaled.

The cannisters are typically made of aluminum and are pressurized to 3–5 bar. The metering valve is the critical delivery component, and these valves are usually designed to dispense (reliably) 25–100 μL of the liquid in the cannister. This is accomplished by the physical design of the metering chamber. Figure 8.5 shows a view of a typical metering valve.

The cannister itself is fitted into an actuator body normally made of plastic. The stem of the metering valve is connected to an expansion

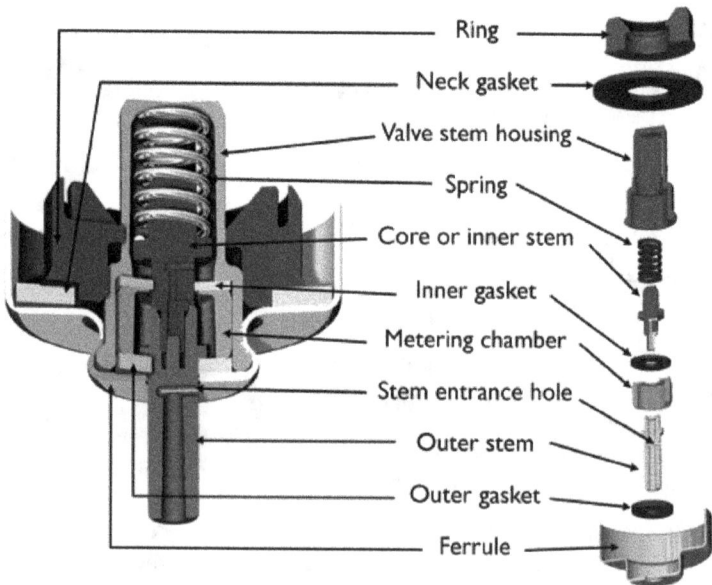

Ring

Neck gasket

Valve stem housing

Spring

Core or inner stem

Inner gasket

Metering chamber

Stem entrance hole

Outer stem

Outer gasket

Ferrule

Figure 8.5: A cross section and exploded view of a typical metering valve from a pMDI. The design of the metering valve is a critical factor in the performance of the pMDI. (Reproduced with permission from the International Society for Aerosols in Medicine [ISAM]).

chamber and when the liquid is forcibly ejected from the metering chamber, it exits the expansion chamber via the nozzle. This is typically 0.4–0.6 mm in diameter, although some smaller designs have been used to facilitate the generation of smaller aerosol droplets. The rapid reduction in pressure of the propellant as it enters the expansion chamber causes it to boil and any liquid exiting via the nozzle is subject to significant shearing forces, promoting droplet formation. A plume of droplets exits the actuator casing and as it travels further, evaporation of any remaining propellant occurs.

The plume generated by the pMDI typically exits the device at a quite high velocity and exists only for a short period of time. In the past, such plumes have been ~5 m/s, 10 cm from the nozzle and with a duration of only 0.2 s. This high-velocity plume presents a considerable challenge in delivering the drug to the lung. If it is sprayed directly into the mouth, unless there is active inspiratory flow, the majority of the plume will simply impact the rear of the mouth cavity. Thus, the correct usage of the device requires a degree of coordination on the part of the patient (press the cannister *just after* you have begun to breathe in), which some cannot achieve. More recent formulations have reduced plume velocity using the HFA propellant to the range of ~2 m/s with a duration of 0.4 s.[7] However, even with these reductions in plume velocity, coordination remains challenging.

pMDIs with breath actuation have been developed and these clearly help with the coordination requirements. In these the device is primed to fire and then the actual delivery only occurs when a pre-defined inspiratory flow rate has been achieved by the patient. This is typically accomplished via a mechanical actuator that is triggered by the negative pressure required to generate the inspiratory flow.

One effective solution to the problem of the rapidly travelling plume is the use of a spacer or a valved holding chamber. This is simply a (typically plastic) chamber with a place to insert the pMDI at one end and a mouthpiece at the other end. In some cases, valves are included to ensure flow directionality. This added volume (150–700 mL) allows the plume generated by the pMDI to decelerate and thus reduces the pharyngeal deposition that can result. The other advantage of a spacer is that the need for appropriate coordination between actuating the pMDI and inspiring is greatly reduced. If the pMDI is actuated early, the aerosol will stay in suspension and can be inspired after actuation. In addition, any particularly large aerosol droplets generated by the pMDI (which would deposit by impaction in the upper airway even with good coordination) tend to deposit in the spacer itself.[8]

One of the obvious disadvantages of the use of a spacer is the cumbersome nature of the device. Thus, while it might be feasible to encourage patients to use these at home, their use outside the home is rare. Further, they are often perceived as cumbersome, require cleaning, and so adherence is often poor.

A recent development is that of the "slow mist" or "soft mist" nebulizer. These pocket-sized devices contain the drug in liquid form and the energy for nebulization comes from hydraulic pressure generated by compressing a spring in the device. The device is primed by compressing the spring (typically by twisting part of the casing), and when actuated by a release button, the metered dose is released via a nozzle assembly, with the energy coming from the compressed spring. While this still requires coordination between the pushing of the release button and inhaling, the aerosol is released over a period of 1.5–2 s and with a much lower plume velocity (~0.8 m/s), reducing the coordination requirement.[7] Such devices have been shown to substantially increase the dose of drug that reaches the lung.

8.2.3 Dry Powder Inhalers

Dry Powder Inhalers (DPIs) differ from pMDIs in that, as their name would suggest, the drug is not dissolved or suspended in the liquid, but rather dispensed directly as a powder. The drug in the form of particles with scales in the micron range and a carrier (typically large lactose particles) are formulated as a dry powder mixture and typically contained in small blister packs for a single dose. The devices to deliver the drug vary greatly in design, but all share a common approach, which is that the drug powder mixture is disaggregated by turbulent flow, the energy for which comes from the inspiratory effort of the

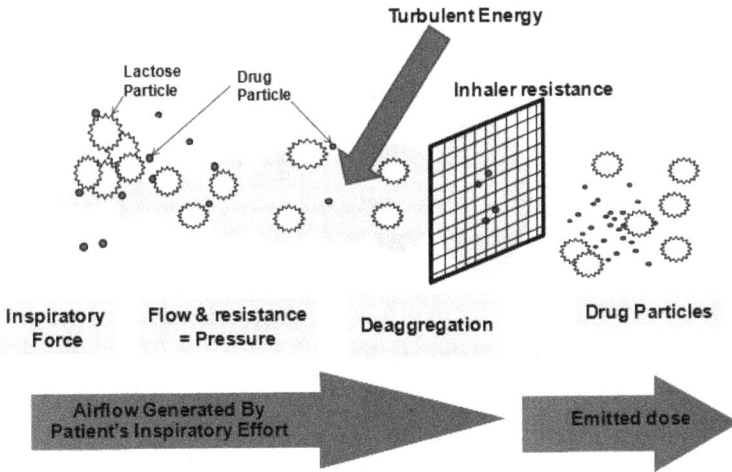

Figure 8.6: The disaggregation of the powder in a DPI is performed through turbulent flow and energy generated by the inspiratory flow of the patient. (Reproduced with permission from the International Society for Aerosols in Medicine [ISAM]).

patient. In order for this to work, the inhaler design includes a resistance element in it so that the inspired flow generates a significant ΔP when inspiration occurs. The drug particles then encounter a turbulent flow regime, which serves to disaggregate them from their settled state in the packaging. Figure 8.6 illustrates the process. As they enter the upper airway, the large lactose particles impact but the small drug particles remain in suspension and are carried into the lung.

This design has the obvious difference from a pMDI of there being no issues associated with coordination (or lack thereof) on the part of the patient. The inhalation itself drives the aerosol cloud generation. However, variations in the design of the devices result in considerable differences in inspiratory resistance, and so in the inspiratory effort required to properly activate the device. This in turn results in variation in the effectiveness of the disaggregation and in turn results in differences in the mass median aerodynamic diameter of the delivered drug. If disaggregation is ineffective and the resultant drug particles are much greater than 5 µm, then these too will impact in the upper airways, especially considering the high inspiratory flow rates required to properly use DPIs.

As a direct consequence of these effects, the dose delivered to the lung is dependent on the peak inspiratory flow rate achieved by the patient.[9,10] Because of differences in device characteristics, there is no universal lower limit on the inspiratory flow required for effective use, but for many devices, this seems to be in the vicinity of 30 L/min (0.5 L/s), a flow rate that most patients can achieve.

Another potential confounder is the inspiratory flow profile. By their design, DPIs release the entire dose of drug at the beginning of inspiration. Thus, if the patient initially inspires slowly, then ineffective disaggregation can occur, compared with a patient who begins the inspiration with a high flow. Thus, just like the case with pMDIs, patient training is important (and often sadly lacking). This is further complicated by the fact that optimal inhaler technique for a pMDI and a DPI differ greatly, further compounding the problems for patients who use both.

8.2.4 *Modern (Smart) Nebulizers*

There has been a considerable pace of development of nebulizers that are "smart" over the last decade or so. There are now numerous models and designs that are on the market.[11,12] In some cases, these are programmable nebulizers allowing a range of settings, and in other cases, these are specifically tailored for the delivery of a specific drug. Any listing of such devices we could make here would inevitably be rapidly out of date. For that reason, we have avoided such an approach and instead have outlined the specific functions or enhancements that these devices employ. It is almost certain this list of functions will increase with time as novel ideas are employed.

Much effort has been devoted to enhancing the efficiency of the drug delivery both through the nebulization process and through improving pulmonary deposition of the aerosolized drug. This includes breath triggering of actuation of the device so that nebulization occurs only when the subject inspires (drug nebulized during expiration clearly does not go into the patient). Controlling where the drug is deposited in the lung is clearly influenced by particles size, and so devices that control particle size (such as vibrating mesh nebulizers) provide a means to target different regions of the lung. Similarly, as described in Chapters 3 and 5, the breathing pattern clearly affects the site of deposition. A high inspiratory flow rate will result in higher upper airway deposition by impaction. Even if the intent is to minimize the upper airway deposition, no amount of particle size generation control will overcome an especially vigorous inspiration on the part of the patient. For that reason, devices that control respiratory flow rates are becoming more common.

In a similar vein, controlling inspiratory volume, coupled with controlled flow rate, and well-defined particle sizes is likely to provide for close to optimal targeting of aerosol deposition. This has even been further advanced to include controlling the aerosol generation within a breath. As discussed in Chapter 5, aerosol boluses placed carefully within a breath provide a means to interrogate distinct portions of the airway tree. Similarly, by controlling the aerosol production within a breath, drug delivery to distinct portions of the airway tree should be possible. For example, if aerosol generation is begun only after the onset of inspiration and terminated after (say) 500 mL of a controlled 1000 mL inspiration, then the aerosol will be followed by a volume of clean air, minimizing central airway deposition (provided flow rate is controlled, see point above). Many of these systems provide feedback to the patient either visually or audibly, but their use requires a considerable degree of patient training.

However "smart" the nebulizers become, it is all for naught if they are not used. Thus, considerable effort is being expended into making the devices both user-friendly and capable of monitoring patient adherence. This is a far from trivial challenge and plays a critical role in deciding whether or not a drug and its associated delivery system will survive. Some inhaled drugs are being presented with their own, specially tailored nebulizer systems (Treprostinil, a pulmonary vasodilator is just one example) that carefully monitor the delivery and usage of the device, and in doing so, provide treatment adherence data to the clinician. History has shown that patient acceptability is critically important, and it is notable that (for example) the first inhaled insulin formulation rollout was hampered, not only by clinically relevant side effects, but also by patient's dislike of the cumbersome nature of the delivery system. The current inhaled insulin delivery system is simple (a DPI, see Section 8.2.3) but whether it becomes well accepted by patients remains to be seen.

References

1. Patton JS, and Byron PR. (2007). Inhaling medicines: Delivering drugs to the body through the lungs. *Nat. Rev. Drug. Discov.* **6**: 67–74.
2. Mak JC, Nishikawa M, and Barnes PJ. (1995). Glucocorticosteroids increase beta 2-adrenergic receptor transcription in human lung. *Am. J. Physiol.* **268**: L41–L46.
3. Laube BL. (2014). The expanding role of aerosols in systemic drug delivery, gene therapy and vaccination: An update. *Transl. Respir. Med.* **2**: 3.
4. Mohanty RR, and Das S. (2017). Inhaled insulin — Current direction of insulin research. *J. Clin. Diagn. Res.* **11**: OE01–OE02.
5. Finlay WH. (2002). *The Mechanics of Inhaled Pharmaceutical Aerosols: An Introduction.* San Diego: Academic Press.
6. Steckel H, and Eskandar F. (2003). Factors affecting aerosol performance during nebulization with jet and ultrasonic nebulizers. *Eur. J. Pharm. Sci.* **19**: 443–455.
7. Hochrainer D, Holz H, Kreher C, Scaffidi L, Spallek M, and Wachtel H. (2005). Comparison of the aerosol velocity and spray duration of Respimat Soft Mist inhaler and pressurized metered dose inhalers. *J. Aerosol. Med.* **18**: 273–282.
8. Marple VA, Roberts DL, Romay FJ, Miller NC, Truman KG, Van Oort M, Olsson B, Holroyd MJ, Mitchell JP, and Hochrainer D. (2003). Next generation pharmaceutical impactor (a new impactor for pharmaceutical inhaler testing). Part I: Design. *J. Aerosol. Med.* **16**: 283–299.
9. Tarsin WY, Pearson SB, Assi KH, and Chrystyn H. (2006). Emitted dose estimates from Seretide Diskus and Symbicort Turbuhaler following inhalation by severe asthmatics. *Int. J. Pharm.* **316**: 131–137.
10. Nadarassan DK, Assi KH, and Chrystyn H. (2010). Aerodynamic characteristics of a dry powder inhaler at low inhalation flows using a mixing inlet with an Andersen Cascade Impactor. *Eur. J. Pharm. Sci.* **39**: 348–354.
11. Brand P, Meyer T, Haussermann S, Schulte M, Scheuch G, Bernhard T, Sommerauer B, Weber N, and Griese M. (2005). Optimum peripheral

drug deposition in patients with cystic fibrosis. *J. Aerosol Med.* **18**: 45–54.

12. Denyer J, Nikander K, and Smith NJ. (2004). Adaptive Aerosol Delivery (AAD) technology. *Expert. Opin. Drug Deliv.* **1**: 165–176.

Chapter 9
Ambient and Indoor Aerosol

9.1 Introduction

Ambient and indoor air always contains aerosol and with each breath, some of this aerosol is deposited in the lung. The lung-deposited aerosol dose and the associated adverse health effects depend on size and chemical composition of the aerosol (Chapters 3 and 10). All of these aerosol parameters are affected by numerous aspects including location, weather conditions, season, type and proximity of aerosol sources.

In this chapter, we present the main natural and anthropogenic (man-made) sources and their contribution to ambient and indoor aerosol concentration, as well as describe their effect on aerosol size range and chemical composition. An overview of typical aerosol mass concentrations is provided for different locations ranging from clean (natural) background conditions over highly polluted urban sites to various indoor conditions. For ambient air, the focus is on urban aerosol due to its prominent role in public health; for both urban and indoor particulate matter (PM) burden, the differences between developed (high-income) and developing (low-income) countries are discussed.

9.2 Ambient Aerosol

Ambient aerosol is characterized by three different size modes referred to as nucleation mode (diameter range 0.005–0.1 μm), accumulation mode (0.1–2 µm) and coarse mode (larger than 2 µm). This trimodal size distribution is often referred to as the Whitby model, since it was introduced by K. T. Whitby in the late 1970s. Each of these modes, which can be described by the characteristic parameters of a lognormal size distribution (here: median aerodynamic diameter (*MMAD*), geometric standard deviation (GSD) and mass concentration (*M*); see Chapter 3), originates from different types of aerosol sources. Each type has very similar mean size and width of the size distribution but is affected by distinctly different mechanisms of aerosol processing and deposition. Table 9.1 provides an overview of these parameters for aerosol mass distributions typically observed at different locations with a focus on clean continental sites (remote continental sites, far away from anthropogenic aerosol sources), average (continental) background conditions (e.g., rural sites with some anthropogenic aerosol), average urban regions (urban sites not in close proximity to strong aerosol sources) and urban sites in the proximity of a freeway.

It is evident from Table 9.1 that *MMAD* and *GSD* (for definition, see Chapter 3) are very similar for each of the (mass-weighted) modes

Table 9.1: Trimodal lognormal volume-/mass-weighted size distribution and the total mass concentration (sum of mass over all modes) of different types of ambient aerosol.

Atmospheric condition	Nucleation mode			Accumulation mode			Coarse mode			Total mass
	MMAD (µm)	GSD	M^a (µg/m³)	*MMAD* (µm)	GSD	M^a (µg/m³)	*MMAD* (µm)	GSD	M^a (µg/m³)	M_{tot} (µg/m³)
Clean continental background	0.03	1.6	0.009	0.35	2.1	2.2	6.0	2.2	7.5	9.7
Average background	0.034	1.7	0.056	0.32	2.0	6.7	6.0	2.2	25.9	32.7
Urban average	0.038	1.8	0.47[b]	0.32	2.2	28.8[b]	5.7	2.2	23.1[b]	42.4
Urban and freeway	0.032	1.7	6.9[b]	0.25	2.0	28.1[b]	6.0	2.1	32.0[b]	67.0

Note: The parameters MMAD, GSD and M represent the mass median aerodynamic diameter, geometric standard deviation and mass concentration of each mode, respectively (Baron and Willeke, 2001, p. 105[1]).

[a] These values were calculated from the volume concentration assuming a particle density of 1.5 g/cm³.

[b] These values were divided by a factor of 2 to account for the cleaner urban conditions today as compared to the 1970s US, which this table is based on (see Figure 9.4).

independent of atmospheric conditions, namely $MMAD = 0.03$–0.04 µm and $GSD = 1.6$–1.8 for the nucleation mode, $MMAD = 0.25$–0.35 µm and $GSD = 2.0$–2.2 for the accumulation mode and $MMAD = 5.7$–6.0 µm and $GSD = 2.1$–2.2 for the coarse mode. Similar consistency is obtained for number and surface area-weighted size distributions, except that the median diameters for each of the three size modes are shifted to smaller diameters. This shift in size distribution can be calculated using the so-called Hatch-Choate equations in the following form[1]:

$$CMD = MMAD/\exp(3 \ln^2 \sigma_g) \qquad (9.1a)$$

$$SAMD = MMAD/\exp(\ln^2 \sigma_g), \qquad (9.1b)$$

where CMD, SAMD and VMAD/MMAD represent the median diameters of the number, surface area, and volume/mass size distribution, respectively. It is important to note that the modal diameters of the volume-weighted and mass-weighted size distribution are identical, as the mass-to-volume conversion factor (particle density) is approximately independent of particle size for most atmospheric conditions. For typical ambient size distributions with a width of $GSD = 2$, SAMD = MMAD/1.6 and CMD = MMAD/4.2, i.e., for surface area and number size distribution, the modal median diameters are shifted to 1.6-fold and 4.2-fold smaller sizes, respectively. For lognormal size distributions, the GSD of the modes are identical for the number, surface area and mass size distribution (see Chapter 3).

As an example of this size shift, the *urban average* mass distribution (see Table 9.1) is converted for each mode into the corresponding number and surface area distribution (Figure 9.1) using the Hatch–Choate equations (Eqs. (9.1a) and (9.1b)) and an assumed spherical particle shape and a constant particle density (1.5 g/cm³), which are both a good approximation for most urban conditions. As seen from Figure 9.1 for the volume-/mass-weighted size distribution, the most relevant size range is 0.1–10 µm with about equal contributions from the accumulation and coarse mode. For the surface area-weighted size distribution, the most relevant size range is shifted to smaller particles (0.015–1 µm) mainly represented by the

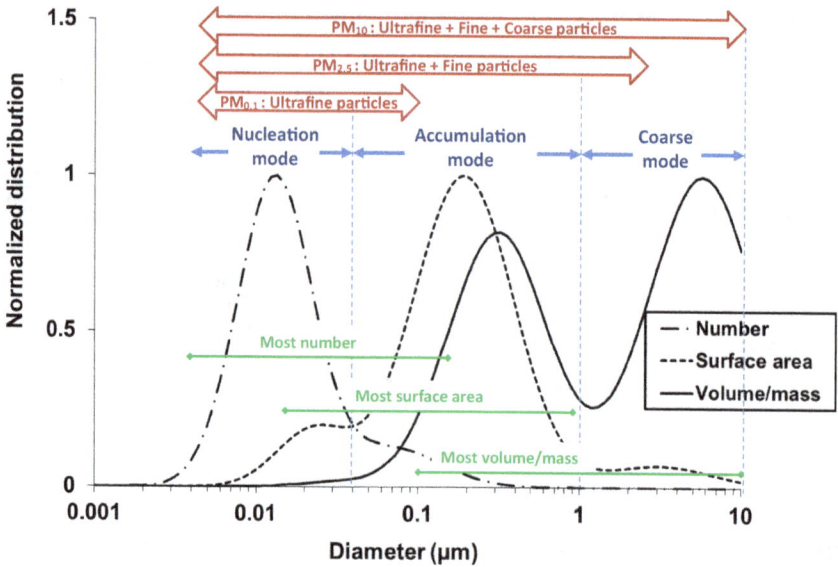

Figure 9.1: The trimodal structure of the (differential) size distribution of urban average aerosol with respect to number ($1/cm^3$), surface area ($\mu m^2/cm^3$) and volume or mass concentration ($\mu m^3/cm^3$ or $\mu g/cm^3$). For ease of presentation, all size distributions are normalized to their respective maximum concentration. According to the Whitby model (blue text/arrows), the number and surface area distribution is dominated by the nucleation and accumulation mode, respectively, while the volume (mass) concentration of urban aerosol consists of about equal contributions from accumulation and coarse mode particles. The most relevant size range for each size distribution is depicted (green text/arrows) and the size range corresponding to ultrafine ($PM_{0.1}$), ultrafine + fine ($PM_{2.5}$) and ultrafine + fine + coarse particles (PM_{10}) is identified (red text/arrows).

accumulation mode (and the larger end of the nucleation mode). The number size distribution is dominated by an even smaller size range of 0.005–0.2 μm, mainly representing the nucleation mode (and the smaller end of the accumulation mode). Thus, the choice of metric determines which size fraction is most relevant that has implications for regulatory measures of ambient PM. For instance, reduction of the particle number concentration requires mitigation of the generation of nucleation mode particles (or ultrafine particles), while mitigation of the PM mass concentration levels requires tighter control of the accumulation and coarse mode particles. This issue will be revisited below when considering the conversion of aerosol *exposure* concentration into lung-deposited aerosol *dose* and associated health effects stratified by number, surface area and volume/mass as dose metric (Chapter 10).

It is important to note that there are different terminologies for the modal structure of ambient aerosol (Figure 9.1). The Whitby model distinguishes three modes (nucleation, accumulation, coarse) based on the origin and mechanism of generation of the particles (see below). Alternatively, a purely size-based approach is widely used, which refers to particles with diameter <0.1 μm, 0.1–2.5 μm and 2.5–10 μm as ultrafine, fine or coarse particles, respectively. Moreover, the abbreviations $PM_{0.1}$, $PM_{2.5}$ and PM_{10} indicate the PM with diameter below 0.1, 2.5 and 10 μm, respectively. It is evident that $PM_{0.1}$ corresponds to the ultrafine particles, $PM_{2.5}$ is the sum of ultrafine and fine particles and PM_{10} is the sum of ultrafine, fine and coarse mode particles (Figure 9.1). From the perspective of the Whitby model, there is a strong resemblance between nucleation (0.004–0.04 μm) and ultrafine (<0.1 μm), accumulation (0.04–1.0 μm) and fine (0.1–2.5 μm), and — of course–(Whitby) coarse (1.0–10 μm) and coarse (2.5–10 μm) mode particles. However, the Whitby model does not impose definite size limits on the three modes but defines the modal structure based on their distinctly different source profiles. All of these issues are illustrated in Figure 9.1.

As mentioned above, the three modes of the Whitby model of ambient aerosol are distinctly different with respect to aerosol sources, processes of aerosol evolution and chemical composition. These issues are summarized, graphically depicted in Figure 9.2 and discussed in the following paragraphs.[1]

Nucleation mode particles (0.004–0.04 μm) originate from natural and anthropogenic gaseous emissions (e.g., from plants, animals and combustion), which include sulfur dioxide (SO_2), nitric oxide/dioxide (NO, NO_2), hydrocarbons (such as methane), ammonia (NH_3), hydrogen sulfide (H_2S) and organics (H–C–O). Nucleation mode particles only occur in the presence of large concentrations of gaseous emissions, which serve as precursors of aerosol. This is typically the case near highways or in close proximity to other highly

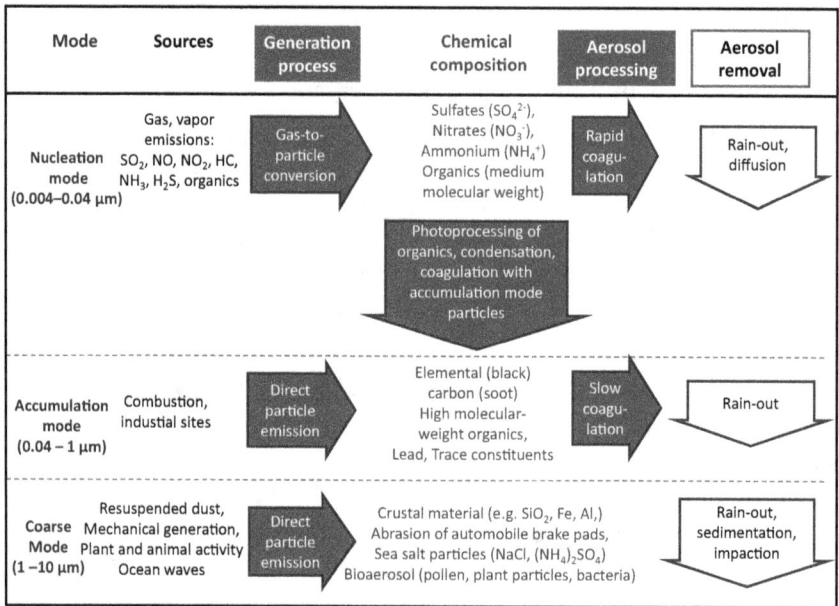

Figure 9.2:   Nucleation, accumulation and coarse mode particles and their specific sources, chemical composition, as well as processes of aerosol formation, evolution and removal.[1,2]

potent combustion sources (e.g., industrial facilities). However, nucleation modes can also appear under extremely clean background conditions. In this case, the required gaseous emissions are provided by forests, which can emit large amounts of gaseous organic compounds. The absence of already existing aerosol — as is typical in clean background conditions — prevents removal of these gases due to condensation onto already existing aerosol. Consequently, under certain temperature and humidity conditions, these gases reach supersaturation and undergo gas-to-particle conversion, resulting in the formation of $0.005–0.02$ µm aerosols containing mainly sulfate, nitrate, ammonium and organics. Due to their small size, nucleation mode particles are highly diffusive, resulting in rapid coagulation and hence fast growth of particles into the 0.05 µm size range. The primary emitted gaseous organic compounds are mainly of low or medium molecular weight. As low molecular weight components are very volatile, only medium molecular weight compounds undergo gas-to-particle conversion. However, in the presence of sunlight, low/medium molecular weight compounds are oxidized into medium/high molecular weight compounds (photoprocessing). This drives the gaseous organic compounds into the nucleation mode and ultimately via agglomeration or condensation on already existing particles into the accumulation mode.

The *accumulation mode* (0.04–1.0 µm) consists of combustion particles of natural (e.g., wildfires) and anthropogenic origin (traffic, heating, etc.), as well as smog (photochemically processed gas-phase emissions) and particles from some industrial activities. Combustion processes always result in the generation of elemental carbon often referred to as black carbon or soot. Depending on fuel type, combustion processes are also associated with substantial emissions of high-molecular-weight organic compounds (precursors of smog) and trace metals such as lead (Pb) and aluminum (Al). As mentioned above, eventually most of the nucleation mode particles will coagulate with accumulation mode particles adding to their organic mass fraction. There is also particle growth due to condensation of organics and self-coagulation processes. However, compared to nucleation mode particles, which undergo rapid coagulation, the coagulation rate of accumulation mode particles is much lower (slow coagulation) due to their larger size.

Coarse mode (1.0–10 µm) particles are generated by processes such as resuspension of crustal dust due to air flow (wind or motion of vehicles) or by mechanical processes such as agricultural, construction or surface mining activities, as well as abrasion of automobile brake pads or other materials exposed to high levels of friction (industrial processes). The coarse mode also contains particles of biologic origin (bioaerosol) such as pollen, plant debris, bacteria, viruses and fungi. Last but not least, sea salt aerosol generated by the breaking of ocean waves contributes to the coarse mode often even in regions not directly located near coastlines (long-range transport). Ultimately, all aerosols are eventually removed from the atmosphere again. The main mechanisms of aerosol removal from the atmosphere are rain-out (capture of aerosol by falling rain drops) and deposition on surfaces due to diffusion (nucleation mode) or sedimentation and impaction (coarse mode).

9.3 Urban Aerosol

The number, surface area and mass size distribution of *urban average* aerosol has been depicted in Figure 9.1. The main sources of urban aerosol include local combustion activities, industrial emissions (e.g., manufacturing industry, waste incineration), resuspended crustal material (e.g., dust, soil), abrasion of brake wear and nonlocal sources transferring aerosols from other regions to urban area, sometimes over thousands of miles apart (Figure 9.2). Depending on location, time, season and atmospheric conditions, the relative contributions of these sources can be quite different.

As an example, Figure 9.3 depicts the annually averaged source profile of urban PM in a central European city.[3] It is evident that about **40%** of the aerosol mass is transported into the city. Thus, even

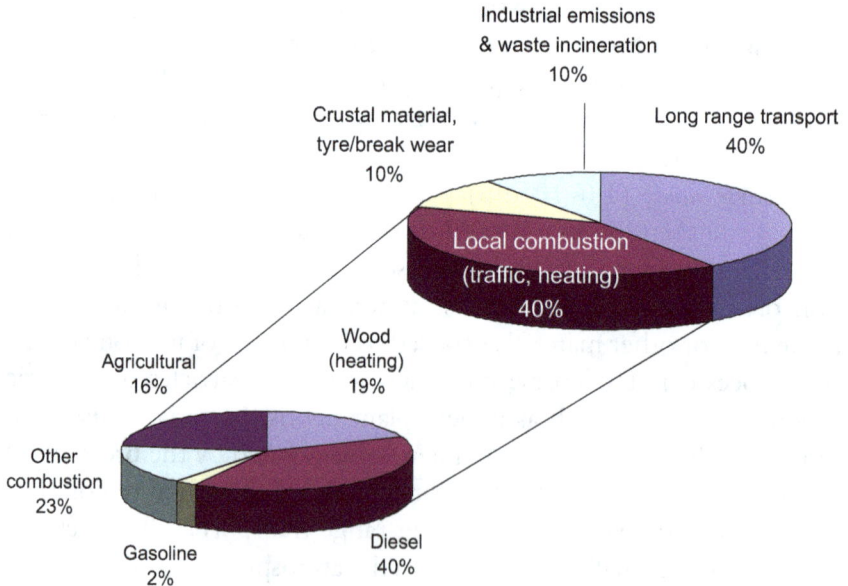

Figure 9.3: Main sources of urban aerosol and their relative contribution to the annual average $PM_{2.5}$ burden of cities in central Europe.[3]

if emissions from the metropolitan region could be reduced to zero, the $PM_{2.5}$ burden would only drop by about a factor of ~2. Thus, even the best PM mitigation strategies can only accomplish a reduction in PM exposure by a factor of ~2. Typically, the main local aerosol sources are related to combustion activities (ca. 40%), which can be further stratified into combustion of diesel (40% of local combustion aerosol), as well as heating (19%), agricultural (16%) and other combustion activities (23%). In comparison to Diesel, gasoline combustion plays only a minor role (2%). The remainder of about 20% of PM is distributed equally amongst crustal material, tyre, and brake wear (10%) and emissions from industrial activities including waste incineration (10%).[3–6]

The detailed chemical composition of ambient aerosol depends on numerous factors including the type and relative contribution of aerosol sources, photochemical processing, residence time in the atmosphere and rain-out or dry aerosol deposition. Table 9.2 presents

Table 9.2: Chemical composition of urban aerosol as compared to rural background aerosol stratified for fine and coarse mode aerosol.

Molecular/atomic compounds	Urban (%)		Rural (%)	
	Fine	Coarse	Fine	Coarse
Sulfate (SO_4^-)	**40.5**	4.1	**50.0**	0
Nitrate (NO_3^+)	0.6	6.7	1.3	0
Ammonium (NH_4^+)	**10.2**	0.7	**9.6**	0
Acidic hydrogen (H^+)	0.2	0.04	0.5	0
Carbon (C)	**18.1**	12.2	13.8	23.2
Aluminum (Al)	0.2	5.2	0.1	3.6
Silicon (Si)	0.5	**14.1**	0.2	19.4
Sulfur (S)	0	0	**15.4**	3.6
Calcium (Ca)	0.4	11.5	0.1	5.7
Iron (Fe)	0.4	2.7	0.1	2.1
Lead (Pb)	1.1	0.5	4.0	0.3
Nitrogen (N), oxygen (O) from organic compounds (and unidentified compounds)	27.8	**42.3**	4.9	**47.5**

Note: The top four contributions are shown in bold letters. (Adapted from Hinds, 1999, p. 314[2]).

an example for the atomic and molecular composition of urban and rural PM_{10} stratified for fine and coarse particle mode particles. It is evident that elemental carbon from combustion sources is among the most important compounds for all cases. Sulfate from sea salt and sulfur-containing fuel combustion (which was still used in the 1980s) is the most relevant compound for fine particles, as well as ammonium (sea salt). Organics compounds also play an important role for all cases except for rural fine-mode particles. Metal compounds are significant contributors to coarse mode particles (mineral dust).

9.4 Global Aerosol Emissions

On a global scale urban, the annual average $PM_{2.5}$ levels are varying widely ranging from <10 µg/m³ to >35 µg/m³ (Figure 9.4). $PM_{2.5}$ typically accounts for 50%–70% of urban PM_{10} in developed countries of the western hemisphere and is often considered the toxicologically most relevant PM fraction in part due to its high contribution to the particle surface area (Figure 9.1), as will be discussed in Chapter 10. The lowest

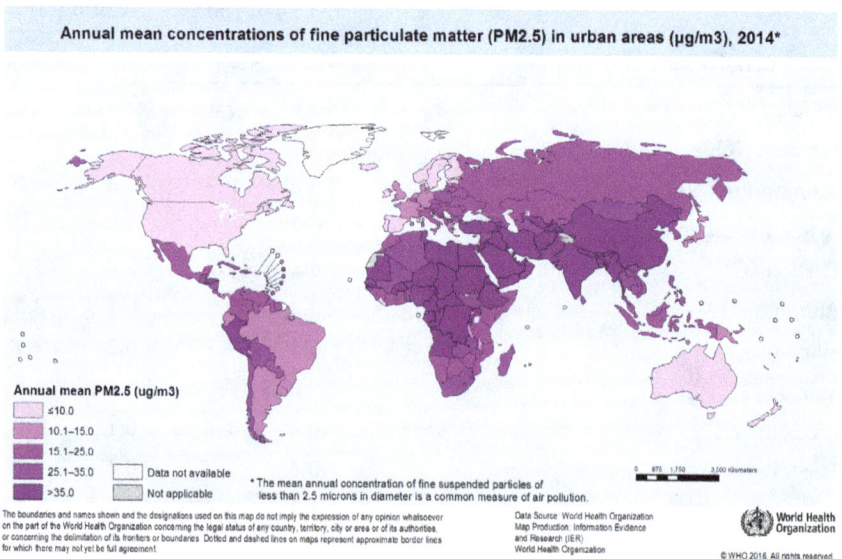

Figure 9.4:   Global map of the annual mean mass concentration of $PM_{2.5}$ in urban regions in 2014.[4]

$PM_{2.5}$ levels of below 10 µg/m³ are found in northern America, some parts of northern and southern Europe (Island, Ireland, Spain, Portugal), as well as in Australia and New Zealand. On the other hand, the most polluted urban areas with $PM_{2.5}$ levels about 35 µg/m³ are currently mainly found in central to north-eastern Africa, the Arabian Peninsula, Turkey, Persia, India and China, as well in a few countries in central and southern America (Guatemala and Peru). In these regions, annual average $PM_{2.5}$ levels much larger than 35 µg/m³ can occur. For instance, for numerous cities in India, exposure levels between 100 and 350 µg/m³ have been reported[7] and among 210 cities in China, values between 11 and 128 µg/m³ have been observed.[8] It is important to note that even for the most polluted urban regions, not only anthropogenic but also natural sources (e.g., wildfires, long-range transport of desert dust) are contributing significantly to the observed PM levels. This issue will be discussed in more detail below.

It is also noteworthy that the trimodal *urban average* mass size distribution given in Table 9.1 represents a $PM_{2.5}$ concentration of 29.3 µg/m³ (sum of nucleation and accumulation mode), which corresponds to the second most highest exposure level (25.1–35.0 µg/ m³) depicted in the global $PM_{2.5}$ map provided by the World Health Organization (WHO, Figure 9.4).

While in some highly polluted areas such as those near freeways or in roadway tunnels, anthropogenic sources may dominate the PM levels, this is not the case on a global scale, where anthropogenic aerosol emissions account for <15% of the total PM burden (Table 9.3). The main natural aerosol sources of ambient PM are deserts and oceans (desert dust, sea salt particles). Forest regions also contribute substantially to ambient PM mainly due to emission of volatile organics, which undergo gas-to-particle conversion and — to a much lesser degree — due to forest fires. The remainder is due to sunlight (photoprocessing of gaseous compounds) and botanical debris. Volcanic eruptions also contribute measurably to the global PM budget. On average, their contribution is below 1%, but occasionally volcanic eruptions can enhance the global PM burden by as much as 100% and result in a global cooling effect. The relatively small contribution of anthropogenic sources to global PM (12.8%) is mainly due to combustion, agricultural and industrial processes, resulting into direct

Table 9.3: Relative contribution of natural and anthropogenic sources to global emission of ambient aerosol mass.

Source	Contribution to global emissions (%)
Natural	
Soil/desert dust	41.7
Sea salt	36.1
Gas-to-particle conversion	5.0
Photochemical processing	1.7
Botanica debris	1.4
Volcanic eruption	0.8
Forest fires	0.6
Total for natural sources	**87.2**
Anthropogenic	
Gas-to-particle conversion	9.2
Direct emissions (e.g., soot or brake pad abrasion)	3.3
Photochemical processing	0.3
Total for anthropogenic emissions	**12.8**

Note: Adapted from Hinds, 1999, p. 305.[2]

particle emissions (3.3%), and gaseous emissions with subsequent gas-to-particle conversion (9.2%) (see Table 9.3).

In light of the high abundance of naturally occurring aerosol, anthropogenic aerosol sources may seem of minor relevance. However, the type and location of aerosol emission are crucial for their impact. Anthropogenic particles from combustion (soot) or industrial activities are typically emitted in or near urban areas where the population density is highest. As these types of particles have been shown to induce adverse health effects, anthropogenic aerosol emissions are a major concern of public health (see Chapter 10). Moreover, anthropogenic aerosol has been shown to affect global warming, although its net effect is currently considered to be relatively small due to competing effects from cooling and heating mechanisms, depending on the type of aerosol and their location of release.

9.5 Indoor Aerosol

Historically, indoor aerosol has received much less attention than ambient aerosol. This is partially due to the fact that ambient aerosol is the driver of important atmospheric and climate phenomena related to global warming. Moreover, ambient aerosol concentrations are measured routinely in thousands of locations worldwide and epidemiological studies have demonstrated strong associations with adverse health effects and ambient PM (see Chapter 10).

However, in developed countries of the western world, people spend about 90% of their time indoors and even in developing countries, indoor exposure levels can be orders of magnitude larger than ambient concentrations. The national human activity pattern survey from 2001 has shown that US people spend about 87% of their time indoors, mostly in residential homes (69%), but also in office and factory buildings (5%), bars and restaurants (2%) and in other indoor environments (11%).[9] Only about 7% and 6% of their time is spent outdoors and in vehicles, respectively. These issues have led to the recognition of indoor aerosol as a potentially important aspect of public health, spurring intensified research on sources and source strengths of indoor aerosol during the past three decades.

In general, indoor aerosol concentrations vary more severely than outdoor (ambient) aerosol. This is a result of the combined effect of the numerous factors that influence indoor aerosol concentration (Figure 9.5). Indoor aerosol is typically closely correlated with outdoor aerosol parameters due to air exchange via infiltration/exfiltration (e.g., not perfectly tight windows) and/or ventilation (active ventilation system or opening of windows). In the absence of indoor aerosol sources, the aerosol concentration in buildings is typically ca. 10%–30% lower than the outdoor aerosol concentration due to deposition of aerosol on walls and other surfaces in the building. This reduction in aerosol concentration is mainly due to the removal of coarse mode particles (2.5–10 µm in diameter), which have the highest settling/deposition rates. As a consequence, the indoor–outdoor correlation of coarse mode particles is typically poor, while it is strong for $PM_{2.5}$ particles. In the presence of active aerosol filtration systems, $PM_{2.5}$ particles are efficiently removed, resulting in even lower indoor

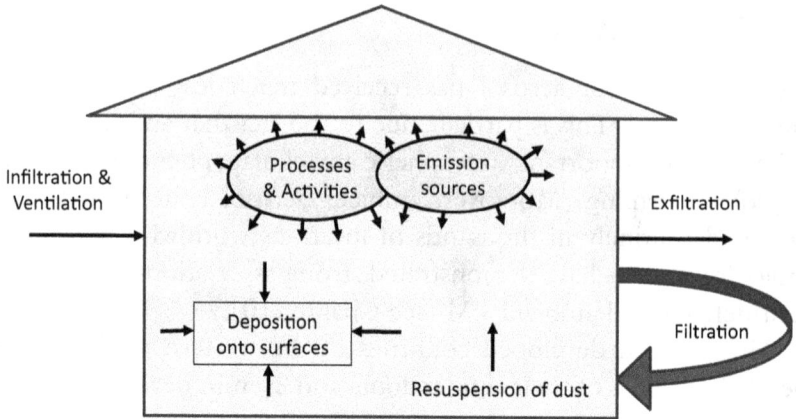

Figure 9.5:   Main factors influencing indoor aerosol concentration. (Adapted from Morawska *et al.* 2017.[11])

aerosol concentrations. On the other hand, in the presence of indoor aerosol sources, elevations in indoor aerosol concentrations can occur and persist for extended periods of time, depending on the ventilation or filtration rate.[10]

During indoor pollution events, the aerosol concentration can exceed outdoor aerosol concentrations by orders of magnitude (>100-fold). Table 9.4 provides an overview of some of the most relevant indoor aerosol sources and their effect on the observed indoor PM_{10} mass concentration. While each individual building and indoor activity is different, leading to differences in peak concentrations and average exposure levels, the listed values represent the upper range of source-specific PM_{10} increase reported in the literature. For residential homes, we distinguish between developed and developing countries representing the <10 $\mu g/m^3$ and >35 $\mu g/m^3$ $PM_{2.5}$ regions depicted in Figure 9.4, respectively. For the former, cigarette smoking and e-cigarette vaping are by far the most potent indoor aerosol sources (500–1300 $\mu g/m^3$) followed by candle burning, vacuum cleaning and frying of food having an at least 5-fold lower effect on PM_{10} than cigarette smoking. Using a cooker hood can substantially reduce aerosol emission during frying down to levels similar to operating a toaster (30 $\mu g/m^3$). Most indoor aerosol sources emit only

Table 9.4: PM$_{10}$ mass concentrations observed for various indoor aerosol sources and associated activities.

Source, activity	PM$_{10}$ mass concentration ($\mu g/m^3$)
Residential (developed countries)	
Cigarette smoking	1300
e-cigarette	500
Candle burning	100
Vacuum cleaner	100
Frying	100
Frying with cooker hood	30
Toaster	30
Residential (developing countries)	
Cooking, heating (with solid fuel)	>1500
Cigarette smoking	1500
Sweeping	1500
Office	
Laser printer	10

Note: These values can vary significantly depending on ventilation, type of appliances and individual (values obtained from Refs. 7, 13–16).

particles below 1 μm (PM$_1$), except for vacuum cleaning (ca. 50% PM$_{1-10}$) and toasters (ca. 100%), which emit ca. 50% and 100% in the PM$_{1-10}$ range, respectively. Hence, the PM$_{10}$ values listed in Table 9.4 correspond to PM$_1$ values, except for vacuum cleaning and toasters. In terms of number, indoor aerosol sources can elevate the particle concentration from typically around 10^3 to as much as $10^{12}/cm^3$. In addition, resuspension of deposited particles by air movement, wiping of surfaces or making bed and folding laundry can also be substantial sources of coarse indoor aerosol, because large particles experience the lowest adhesion forces to surfaces, allowing them to become airborne by wind activity or vibration. Another important but less-well characterized source of indoor aerosol relates to bioaerosols such as bacteria, viruses and fungi. The main indoor sources of bioaerosols are humans, pets, plants, plumbing systems, heating/ventilation/

air-conditioning systems, mold, dust resuspension and the outdoor environment.[12]

In residential homes of developing countries, cigarette smoking is among the top pollution sources only exceeded by cooking at (semi-) open fireplaces with solid fuels such as wood or agricultural produce, often in poorly ventilated kitchens. Cooking- and heating-induced PM_{10} exposure levels can be substantially reduced, if liquid fuels are provided (e.g., kerosene, liquefied petroleum gas) or by improving ventilation near the oven or fireplace.[7] Sweeping of the floor can resuspend large amounts of coarse particles, resulting in similar PM_{10} exposure levels as observed for cooking, heating or smoking of cigarettes.

In contrast to outdoor aerosol, and in spite of the severe effect of indoor aerosol on the overall PM burden, indoor aerosol exposure levels in residential homes are currently not regulated except for occupational settings, as will be discussed in Chapter 12.

References

1. Baron PA, and Willeke K. (2001). *Aerosol Measurement*. New York: Wiley Interscience.
2. Hinds WC. (1999). *Aerosol Technology*. New York: Wiley-Interscience publications.
3. Vallius M. (2005). Characteristics and sources of fine particulate matter in urban air. Ph.D. Thesis. Department of Environmental Sciences, University of Kuopio, Kuopio, Finland, p. 79.
4. WHO. (2016). Ambient Air Pollution Data, Information Evidence and Research (IER) of World Health Organisation (WHO). https://www.who.int/phe/publications/air-pollution-global-assessment/en/, Accessed 13 June 2019.
5. Putaud JP, Raes F, Van Dingenen R, Bruggemann E, Facchini MC, Decesari S, Fuzzi S, Gehrig R, Huglin C, Laj P, Lorbeer G, Maenhaut W, Mihalopoulos N, Müller K, Querol X, Rodriguez S, Schneider J, Spindler G, ten Brink H, Torseth K, and Wiedensohler A. (2004). European aerosol phenomenology — 2: Chemical characteristics of particulate matter at kerbside, urban, rural and background sites in Europe. *Atmos. Environ.* **38**: 2579–2595.

6. Putaud JP, Van Dingenen R, Alastuey A, Bauer H, Birmili W, Cyrys J, Flentje H, Fuzzi S, Gehrig R, Hansson HC, Harrison RM, Herrmann H, Hitzenberger R, Huglin C, Jones AM, Kasper-Giebl A, Kiss G, Kousa A, Kuhlbusch TAJ, Loschau G, Maenhaut W, Molnar A, Moreno T, Pekkanen J, Perrino C, Pitz M, Puxbaum H, Querol X, Rodriguez S, Salma I, Schwarz J, Smolik J, Schneider J, Spindler G, ten Brink H, Tursic J, Viana M, Wiedensohler A, and Raes F. (2010). A European aerosol phenomenology — 3: Physical and chemical characteristics of particulate matter from 60 rural, urban, and kerbside sites across Europe. *Atmos. Environ.* **44**: 1308–1320.

7. Pant P, Guttikunda SK, and Peltier RE. (2016). Exposure to particulate matter in India: A synthesis of findings and future directions. *Environ. Res.* **147**: 480–496.

8. Lin YL, Zou JL, Yang W, and Li CQ. (2018). A review of recent advances in research on PM$_{2.5}$ in China. *Int. J. Environ. Res. Public Health* **15**: E438.

9. Klepeis NE, Nelson WC, Ott WR, Robinson JP, Tsang AM, Switzer P, Behar J, Hern S, and Engelmann W. (2001). The national human activity pattern survey (NHAPS): A resource for assessing exposure to environmental pollutants. *J. Expo. Anal. Environ. Epidemiol.* **11**: 231–252.

10. Diapouli E, Eleftheriadis K, Karanasiou AA, Vratolis S, Hermansen O, Colbeck I, and Lazaridis M. (2011). Indoor and outdoor particle number and mass concentrations in Athens. Sources, sinks and variability of aerosol parameters. *Aerosol Air Qual. Res.* **11**: 632–642.

11. Morawska L, Ayoko GA, Bae GN, Buonanno G, Chao CYH, Clifford S, Fu SC, Hanninen O, He C, Isaxon C, Mazaheri M, Salthammer T, Waring MS, and Wierzbicka A. (2017). Airborne particles in indoor environment of homes, schools, offices and aged care facilities: the main routes of exposure. *Environ. Int.* **108**: 75–83.

12. Prussin AJ, and Marr LC. (2015). Sources of airborne microorganisms in the built environment. *Microbiome.* **3**: 78.

13. Abidin NZ, Abidin EZ, Zulkifli A, Karuppiah K, Ismail SNS, and Nordin ASA. (2017). Electronic cigarettes and indoor air quality: A review of studies using human volunteers. *Rev. Environ. Health.* **32**: 235–244.

14. Karrasch S, Simon M, Herbig B, Langner J, Seeger S, Kronseder A, Peters S, Dietrich-Gümperlein G, Schierl R, Nowak D, and Jörres RA. (2017). Health effects of laser printer emissions: A controlled exposure study. *Indoor Air* **27**: 753–765.

15. Colbeck I, Nasir ZA, and Ali Z. (2010). The state of ambient air quality in Pakistan — A review. *Environ. Sci. Pollut. Res. Int.* **17**: 49–63.
16. Colbeck I, Nasir ZA, and Ali Z. (2010). Characteristics of indoor/outdoor particulate pollution in urban and rural residential environment of Pakistan. *Indoor Air* **20**: 40–51.

Chapter 10
Adverse Health Effects of Aerosols

10.1 Introduction

Inhaled aerosols (or particulate matter, PM) depositing in the lung (see Chapters 3, 5 and 9.1.3) can induce either therapeutic (see Chapters 7 and 8) or detrimental effects on human health depending on their composition. Among the many pollutants in our homes, at work and in the ambient environment, inhaled ambient particles — often referred to as PM — are considered the most lethal environmental contaminant accounting for about half of the premature deaths worldwide (51%) associated with pollutants.[1] On the other hand, therapeutic aerosols containing drugs are widely used for treating diseases of the lung (Chapters 7 and 8). The key to understanding aerosol-related health effects lies in unraveling the link between aerosol exposure and associated adverse health effects.

A simplified, schematic depiction of the complex network of interactions relating aerosol exposure to health risks is depicted in Figure 10.1. Inhaled air typically contains a certain mass concentration ($\mu g/m^3$) of aerosol particles varying in size, shape, density and chemical composition. The exact characteristics of this aerosol depend on a complex matrix of influencing factors such as the type, strength and location of the aerosol sources (e.g., traffic-related combustion, household activities, engineered nanomaterials, etc.), meteorological conditions (temperature, humidity, wind direction), topography (e.g., valley, planes), photochemical processing (degree of sunshine) and many other factors (see Chapter 9). Upon inhalation, some of the

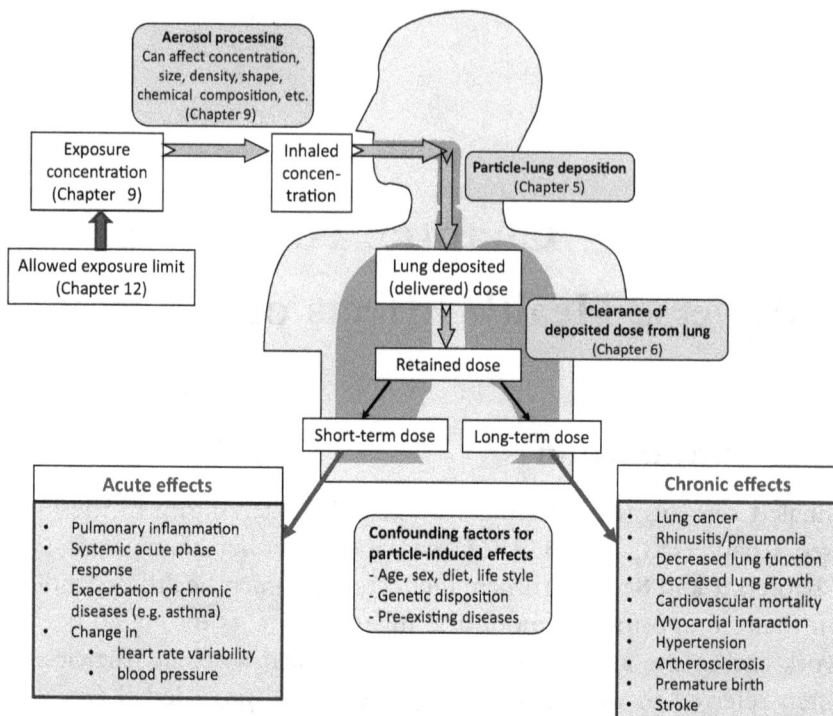

Figure 10.1:　Schematic depiction of key aspects connecting aerosol exposure with lung-delivered particle dose and associated adverse health effects.

aerosol will deposit on the lung tissue and some will be exhaled without depositing in the lung. The lung-deposited aerosol dose depends mainly on the physical and chemical aerosol properties and the respiratory parameters such as breathing frequency and tidal volume (volume of air inhaled per breath), which mainly depends on age, sex, health status and level of physical activity (Chapter 5). The deposition of aerosol particles on the lung tissue may not necessarily result in adverse health effects, because the lung is able to defend itself. A fraction of the deposited aerosol dose is removed from the lung by mucociliary clearance (ca. one third, within hours) and taken up by alveolar macrophages (ca. one third, within months); the remainder (ca. one third) is permanently retained in the lung (see Chapter 6). In spite of these defense mechanisms of the lung, inhaled aerosol can induce both short-term (acute) and long-term (chronic) health effects not only in the lung but also in the cardiovascular system and other organs such as the brain and the reproductive system (see Figure 10.1). It is important to note that not only aerosol dose, but many other factors are also known to affect the disease outcome. Among these so-called confounding factors are age, sex, diet, life style (e.g., physical activity, alcohol consumption, cigarette smoking), preexisting diseases, and genetic predisposition.

In light of the high degree of complexity associated with linking aerosol exposure to adverse health effects, it is necessary to combine data, methods and insights from different scientific disciplines. This chapter gives an overview on (1) determination of the lung-delivered aerosol dose for urban conditions, (2) adverse health effects related to inhaled aerosol, and (3) aerosol-related health risks from the perspectives of epidemiology, clinical studies and toxicology.

10.2 Linking Aerosol Concentration to Lung-Deposited Dose

Ambient or occupational air quality monitoring stations typically report aerosol exposure levels in terms of mass or number concentration, i.e., mass or number of particles per volume of air ($\mu g/m^3$ or $1/cm^3$) (see Chapter 9). As mentioned above, airborne particles can only induce adverse health effects, if they are deposited on the lung epithelium (Figure 10.1). Thus, not aerosol exposure levels, but lung-deposited aerosol dose is the most relevant measure for aerosol-induced health effects. While historically mass and to a lesser degree number are the most widely used dose metrics, it will be shown below that surface area is the toxicologically most relevant dose metric for biopersistent particles, i.e., particles such as soot that are non- or poorly degradable by biological processes (see Chapter 10.3.3).

The lung-deposited aerosol dose mainly depends on the aerosol concentration of the inhaled air. For practical reasons, the aerosol concentration at the point of inhalation is difficult to determine. Hence, one often relies on the (mean) exposure concentration measured at a nearby location. As described in Equation (Eqs. (10.1) lung-deposited dose is then calculated by accounting for the fractional deposition of the inhaled aerosol (*Dep*) and the inhaled air volume ($\dot{V}_{inh} \cdot t_A$) and the surface area of the (human) lung (A_{lung}). Hence, the so-called normalized lung-deposited aerosol dose $Dose_{dep}$, which can be expressed as lung-deposited particle mass per surface area of the lung epithelium, can be calculated from

$$Dose_{dep} = E \cdot Dep \cdot \dot{V}_{inh} \cdot t_A / A_{lung} \qquad (10.1)$$

$Dose_{dep}$ Cumulative lung-deposited dose (mass, surface area, number) normalized to a relevant lung scaling factor (M_{lung}, A_{lung}, N_{lung} — see below).

E Mean exposure concentration at point of inhalation (Chapter 9)

Dep Mean probability for inhaled particles to deposit in the lung (depends among other parameters on particle size; Chapter 5)

$\dot{V}_{inh}$ Mean inhaled air volume per time (typically 25 m³/day; for details, see Table 10.1)

t_A Total exposure (inhalation) time

A_{lung} Surface area of lung epithelium (adult lung: 100 m²); in addition, other lung normalization parameters such as number of exposed cells (N_{lung} = 5.6×10¹⁰ epithelial cells) or mass of lung (M_{lung} =1.3 kg) may be useful.

The advantage of normalizing the lung-deposited dose to a lung-specific scaling factor is allometric scaling, i.e., the determination of equivalent doses for different exposed organisms. Obviously, a dose that is toxic for humans may be even more or less toxic for smaller or larger animals. To account for these species-specific differences, it is useful to normalize the deposited dose to a biologically relevant scaling factor such as body weight or — for inhaled substances more relevant — lung-specific parameters such as surface area of lung epithelium (adult lung: 100 m²), number of exposed cells (N_{lung} = 5.6 × 10¹⁰ epithelial cells) or mass of lung (M_{lung} = 1.3 kg).

For humans, some typical values of the average inhaled air flow rate $\dot{V}_{inh}$ are presented in Table 10.1. Due to particle clearance mechanisms such as mucociliary or macrophage clearance, only ca. 30% of the deposited dose remains in the lung for good (Chapter 6), which

Table 10.1: Representative values of inhaled air flow rate $\dot{V}_{inh}$ (calculated as the product of respiratory frequency [f] and tidal volume [V_T]) for healthy, middle-aged male and female breathing at different activity levels.[2]

	$\dot{V}_{inh}$ (m³/h)	f (breath/min)	V_T (L)
Female			
Rest (sitting)[a]	0.39	14	0.46
Light exercise[a]	1.25	21	0.99
Heavy exercise[b]	2.7	33	1.36
Male			
Rest (sitting)[a]	0.54	12	0.75
Light exercise[a]	1.5	20	1.25
Heavy exercise[b]	3	26	1.92

Note: Typically, ca. 25 m³ of air is inhaled during 1 day.
[a]Nose breathing.
[b]Mouth breathing.

is important for conversion of the lung-deposited dose into long-term retained dose. It is noteworthy that the deposited dose ($Dose_{dep}$) mainly depends on particle size and inhaled air volume ($\dot{V}_{inh} \cdot t_A$), which is related to activity level. As seen from Table 10.1, $\dot{V}_{inh}$ is about 6-fold larger for heavy exercise than for resting conditions and according to Eq. (10.1), this results in a ca. 6-fold higher lung-deposited dose. The typically assumed daily inhaled air volume of 25 m³ lies between the corresponding 24 h values for resting and light exercise conditions.

The alveolar region of the lung is typically considered the most vulnerable part of the lung, because it is not protected by the mucus layer (Chapter 2). Assuming a typical size distribution of urban PM as provided in Table 9.1 and applying the ICRP lung deposition model (Chapter 5), the size-resolved lung deposited dose is calculated for the alveolar region of the lung in terms of number, surface area (assumed spherical particles) and mass (assumed particle density of 1.5 g/cm³) as the dose metric. It is evident from Figure 10.2 (panel A) that depending on the dose metric, different segments of the aerosol size distribution dominate the alveolar lung-deposited dose. For

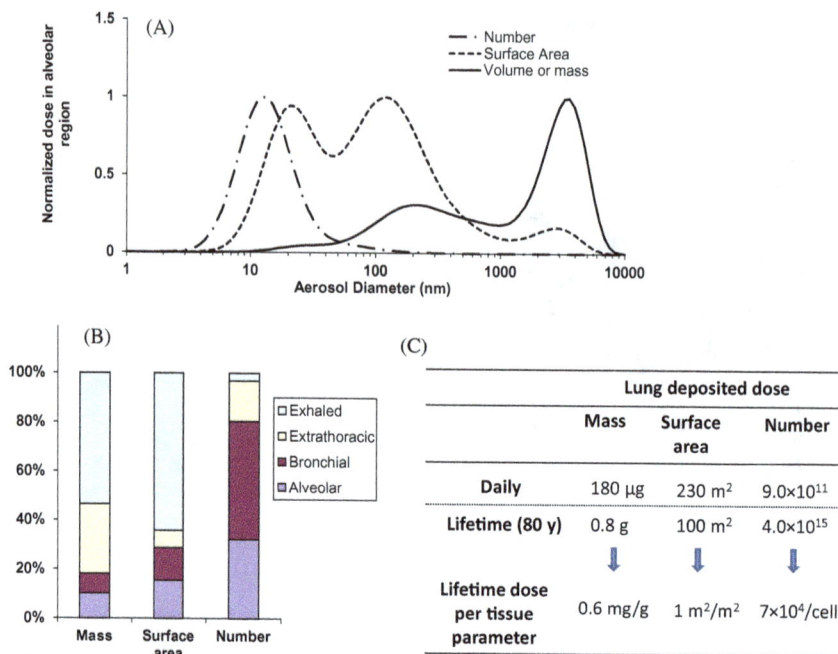

Figure 10.2: Lung-deposited PM dose for urban PM exposure considering number, surface area and mass (or volume) as dose metric. The underlying assumptions of this estimate are described in the text. Panel (A) Size-resolved lung-deposited dose in the alveolar region. For comparison, all curves have been normalized to their respective maximum. It is evident that number, surface area and mass doses are dominated by sub-100 nm, sub-300 nm and above-300 nm aerosol, respectively. Panel (B) Exhaled and regionally deposited fraction of inhaled urban aerosol. Panel (C) Normalized daily and lifetime doses deposited in the total lung (bronchial and alveolar region) in terms of mass, surface area and number according to Eq. 10.1.

number, surface area and mass, the sub-100 nm, sub-300 nm and above-300 nm size segments provide the largest contribution to lung burden, respectively, as represented by the area under the curve in Figure 10.2 (panel A).

Figure 10.2 (panel B) presents the fractions of inhaled particles deposited in different regions of the lung, which again depend on the choice of dose metric. The alveolar deposition fraction increases from 10%, over 15% to 30% for mass, surface area and number dose, respectively. Interestingly, less than 5% of the inhaled aerosol is exhaled in terms of number, but more than 50% is exhaled in terms of surface area and mass. Thus, using the biologically most relevant dose metric is essential for developing the most effective strategies for mitigation of health risks. If indeed particle surface area is the most relevant dose metric, reduction of sub-300 nm aerosol, which is similar to the so-called ultrafine size range (sub-100 nm), would be expected to be an effective mitigation strategy of PM-induced health risks.

Figure 10.2 (panel C) lists the lifetime doses accumulated in the bronchial and alveolar region of lung for urban PM conditions (near freeways) as typically encountered in US and European cities, where we assumed that (1) only 30% of the lung-deposited dose is retained in the lung due to clearance mechanisms, (2) 50% of urban PM is biopersistent (nonbiodegradable), and (3) urban average PM exposure levels and size distributions as reported in Table 9.1 were used (and Hatch-Choate equations were applied; see Eq. 9.1). This yields lifetime doses of 0.6 mg PM per gram of lung, 1 cm^2 PM per cm^2 of lung surface area and 70,000 particles per epithelial cell of the lung. This implies that at the end of our lives, the surface area of the lung-deposited PM is the same as that of the lung (ca. 100 m^2). Of course, under more polluted conditions, these values can be substantially higher.

10.3 Evidence for PM-Induced Health Effects

Evidence for aerosol related, PM induced adverse health effects originates mainly from epidemiology and toxicology and to a lesser degree from clinical studies. Results from these different disciplines are complementary as their respective strengths partially compensate inherent shortcomings of studies from the other disciplines.

Epidemiology investigates statistical correlations between PM exposure and medical records of a large group of people (Figure 10.3). It is found that elevated PM exposure levels are associated with enhanced disease prevalence. These kinds of correlations provide a quantitative assessment of health risks associated with aerosol exposure levels. However, it is important to note that statistical correlations do not necessarily indicate a causal link. This is generally true

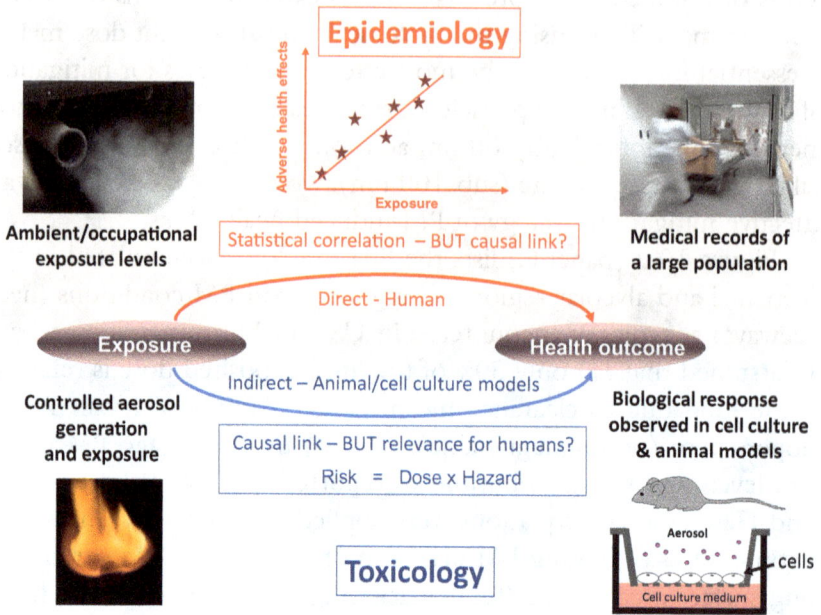

Figure 10.3:   Schematic depiction of the epidemiologic and toxicology approach to studying aerosol-related health effects. While epidemiology leverages human data, it relies on statistical correlations, which are not necessarily an indication of causality. On the other hand, toxicological studies allow for in-depth studies of causal links between aerosol dose and health effects, but only in model organisms, not in humans.

and becomes evident, if we consider an example from economy. It can be shown that there is a strong correlation between the price of train tickets and restaurant prices, but there is no direct causal link between the cost of moving trains and of cooking food, i.e., lowering the price of train tickets would not affect restaurant prices and vice versa. This type of statistical correlation, but not a necessary causal link is often observed in complex systems where a multitude of factors influence certain parameters. For epidemiological studies on PM-induced health risks, this stresses the need for identification and elimination of *so-called* confounding factors, i.e., known risk factors of disease that are correlated with PM exposure but not linked causally. For PM exposure, such confounding factors include cigarette smoking, noise exposure and income level. Each of these parameters is recognized as risk factor for health and at least for one of them — noise — is often strongly correlated with traffic-induced PM exposure, but not causally linked to PM. As low-cost housing is often available in more polluted areas, income level is also a known confounder of PM-related health effects as well as cigarette smoking. Hence, the incidental correlation between a confounding factor and PM exposure levels will induce a bias in the PM-related health effect correlation. Careful identification and quantitative assessment of the effect of confounding factors are often difficult, but a prerequisite for reliable assessment of PM-induced health risks based on epidemiological data.

Toxicology offers an alternative approach to studying PM-induced health effects (Figure 10.3). In toxicology, dose-dependent toxicological response is monitored in model organisms (e.g., animal or cell models) after controlled PM exposure. Careful study design provides minimization of bias due to confounding factors and direct insight into molecular and cellular mechanisms involved in PM-induced toxicological responses. However, translation of these results from model organisms to human exposure scenarios is often challenging due to biological differences between humans and model organisms (Figure 10.3). To some degree, this translational gap can be alleviated by clinical PM exposure studies, where humans are exposed to, e.g., diesel exhaust aerosol. However, these studies are scarce and can only be performed under low dose conditions without severe health responses due to ethical considerations.

Consequently, research on PM-induced health effects relies on combined insights from epidemiology, short-term clinical studies and dedicated toxicological studies with cell and/or animal models.

10.3.1 *Epidemiological Evidence*

Most of the epidemiologic evidence for PM-induced health effects is derived from case-control, cohort or intervention studies. Due to a lack of information on lung-deposited PM dose in the general population, epidemiological studies rely on PM concentration as surrogate for lung-deposited dose.

10.3.1.1 *Types of epidemiological studies*

Case-control studies are retrospective. Two groups of people are defined, which are identical in all aspects except for the outcome of interest (e.g., specific disease is diagnosed or not). By tracing back PM exposure levels experienced by the two groups, one can assess whether there is a statistically significant correlation between PM exposure and disease prevalence. Case-control studies can provide fast results and are cheaper to perform than most other epidemiological studies. The fact that the analysis is retrospective allows rare diseases or diseases with long latency periods to be investigated, but — on the other hand — makes them more prone to biases such as recall bias, i.e., the systematic difference in how the two groups may recall past events (detrimental effects are more likely to be reported than less-severe effects). In addition, matching both groups with respect to all confounding factors (e.g., age, sex, noise, cigarette consumption) is often difficult, as some confounding factors may not even be known.

Most of the epidemiological information on PM-induced health risks is based on *cohort studies*, which rely on a large population base followed up over a long period of time. Cohort studies can be retrospective or prospective. It is noteworthy that retrospective cohort studies are *not* the same as case-control studies. In *retrospective* cohort studies, already existing medical records from a large population base are stratified retrospectively for exposure levels. If morbidity or mortality increases with PM exposure levels, PM exposure represents a risk factor. In the more commonly performed *prospective* cohort studies, people are recruited into a cohort regardless of their exposure or outcome status. This is one of their important strengths. The study then follows these participants for a defined period of time to assess the development of the outcome/disease of interest and its correlation with PM exposure. Cohort studies are good for assessing prognosis, risk factors and harm. Similar to case-control studies, the effects of confounding factors need to be considered. Another important consideration is attrition. If a significant number of participants are not followed up (dropped out or died), then this may affect the validity of the study. Not only does it decrease the study's statistical power, but there may be an attrition bias in the result, i.e., a significant difference between the groups, which did and did not complete the study. Cohort studies allow assessment of the effect of PM exposure on different diseases. Additionally, they are good for rare exposures occurring, e.g., after an industrial accident. However, cohort studies can be expensive and time-consuming, especially if a long follow-up period is chosen or the disease itself is rare or has a long latency.

Finally, *intervention studies* present a powerful tool for the assessment of PM-induced health risks. In case of a drastic change in exposure scenario occurring at a well-defined time point, changes in the medical records prior and after this event provide insight into both causal links and magnitude of the effect of the specific exposure scenario. Historically, such "drastic" events have been the end-of-lifetime of certain industrial sites,[3] the abolishment of coal burning in certain cities and more recently, the drastic reduction in car traffic during the Olympic Games in Beijing, China, in 2008.[4] The advantage of intervention studies is that large, sudden changes in PM exposure are associated with similarly pronounced changes in health status. These can be studied on a relatively small and readily monitored fraction of the population. This offers excellent statistical power and often insight into mechanisms of disease associated with PM exposure.

10.3.1.2 *Results of epidemiological studies*

Epidemiological studies have shown associations between PM exposure and numerous health effects (Figure 10.1). Pulmonary diseases include not only lung cancer, rhinitis/pneumonia, decreased lung function and reduced lung growth, but also cardiovascular effects such as myocardial infarction, elevated blood pressure (hypertension), atherosclerosis and cardiovascular mortality and even premature birth and stroke. In addition, acute effects have been observed such as pulmonary inflammation, exacerbation of chronic pulmonary diseases such as asthma and systemic and cardiovascular effects such as acute phase response (enhanced serum lipid concentration and changes in heart rate variability and in blood pressure).[1,5]

Often the detrimental effect of some type of disease or pollution on human health is expressed in terms of change in life expectancy, premature deaths or disability-adjusted life years (DALY). The life expectancy is the population averaged age at death. The number of premature deaths refers to the increase of deaths for any given age group as compared to a reference population not affected by the disease or pollution type under investigation. The DALY is a measure of overall disease burden combining the concepts of mortality and morbidity into a single metric as it adds the Years of Life Lost (YLL) due to premature death and the equivalent Years Lost due to Disabilities (YLD), which accounts for the reduced quality of life during the years of disease. DALY can be calculated from

$$\text{DALY} = \text{YLL} + \text{YDL}, \tag{10.2}$$

where $\text{YLL} = N \times L$ and $\text{YDL} = D \times DW \times LD$.

Thus, YLL is the product of the number of deaths (N) and the remaining standard life expectancy at the age of death in years (L). Similarly, YDL is the product of the number of disabled people (D), disability weight (DW) and average duration of the case until remission or death in years (LD). These disability weighing factors are regularly updated by the Global Burden of Disease Study and the World Health Organization (WHO).[6] For instance, acute myocardial infarction, one of the main PM-induced causes of death, has a disability weighing factor of 0.439, i.e., for 10 years of life with this disease, the DALY count increases by 4.39 years.

The best evidence exists for PM-induced health effects exists for $PM_{2.5}$, the mass concentration of all PM with a diameter smaller than 2.5 μm (often also referred to as fine PM fraction).[7] It has been shown that the life expectancy in more than 50 different counties and metropolitan areas throughout the United States is well correlated with $PM_{2.5}$. As seen from Figure 10.4 in regions with average $PM_{2.5}$ values near 10 μg/m^3, the average life expectancy based on data from 1978–1982, was about 76 years. For more polluted regions, life

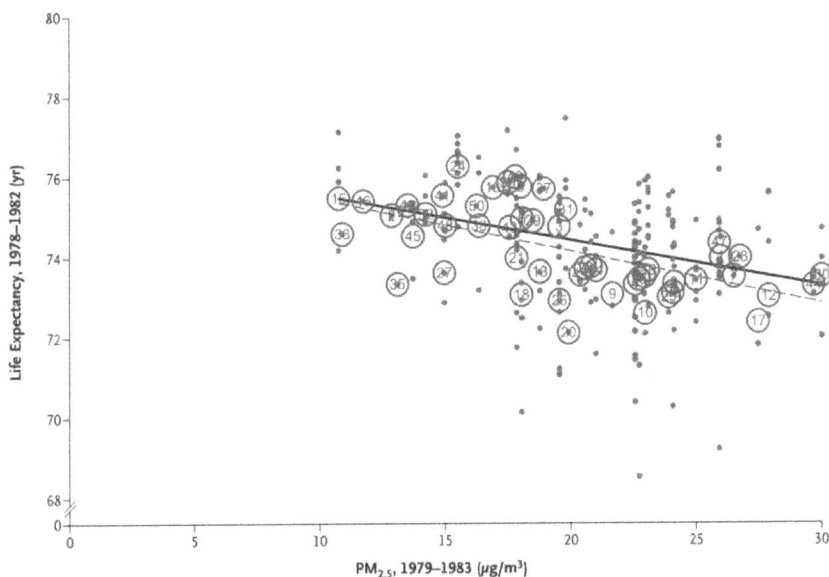

Figure 2. **Cross-sectional life expectancies for 1978–1982, plotted against PM$_{2.5}$ concentrations for 1979–1983.** Dots and circles labeled with numbers represent population-weighted mean life expectancies at the county level and the metropolian-area level, respectively. The solid and broken lines represent regression lines with the use of county-level and metropolitan-area–level observations, respectively. The metropolitan areas are coded by number as follows: 1 — Akron, Ohio; 2 — Albuquerque, New Mexico; 3 — Allentown, Pennsylvania; 4 — Atlanta; 5 — Boise, Idaho; 6 — Boston; 7 — Buffalo, New York; 8 — Charlotte, North Carolina; 9 — Charleston, West Virginia; 10 — Chicago; 11 — Cincinnati; 12 — Cleveland; 13 — Dallas; 14 — Dayton. Ohio; 15 — Denver; 16 — El Paso, Texas; 17 — Gary, Indiana; 18 — Houston; 19 — Indianapolis; 20 — Jersey City, New York City; 21 — Kansas City, Missouri; 22 — Little Rock, Arkansas; 23 — Los Angeles; 24 — Minneapolis; 25 — New York City; 26 — Norfolk, Virginia; 27 — Oklahoma City; 28 — Philadelphia; 29 — Phoenix, Arizona; 30 — Pittsburgh; 31 — Portland, Oregon; 32 — Providence, Rhode Island; 33 — Pueblo, Colorado; 34 — Raleigh, North Carolina; 35 - Reno, Nevada; 36 — St. Louis; 37 — San Diego, California; 38 — San Francisco; 39 — Salt Lake City; 40 — San Jose, California; 41 — Seattle; 42 — Spokane, Washington; 43 — Springfield, Massachusetts; 44 — Steubenville, Ohio; 45 — Tampa, Florida; 46 — Topeka, Kansas; 47 — Washington, D.C.; 48 — Wichita; 49 — Wilmington, Delaware; 50 — Worcester, Massachusetts; 51 — Youngstown, Ohio, PM$_{2.5}$ denotes particulate matter with an aerodynamic diameter less than or equal to 2.5 μm.

Figure 10.4: Cross-sectional life expectancies for 1978–1982, plotted against PM$_{2.5}$ concentrations for 1979–1983 in 51 counties and metropolitan areas of the United States (Reprinted with permission from Ref. 8.).

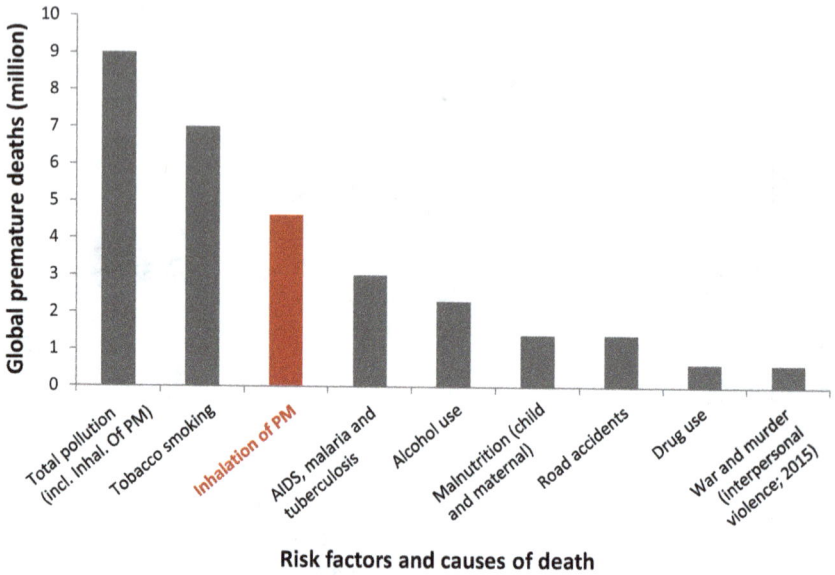

Figure 10.5:   Global estimated premature deaths by relevance of risk factor and cause of death in 2015 (Adapted from Ref. 1.).

expectancy decreases linearly with increasing $PM_{2.5}$, reaching 73 years for $PM_{2.5}$ values near 30 $\mu g/m^3$.

On a global scale, inhalation of PM is amongst the largest risk factors to human health, second only to cigarette smoking (Figure 10.5). In 2015, all forms of pollution (e.g., soil, water, air including inhalation of PM) caused 9 million premature deaths and more than half of this (4.6 million) can be attributed to inhalation of PM (4.2 and 0.4 million to ambient and occupational PM, respectively). Other risk factors such as cigarette smoking (7 million) as well as aids, malaria and tuberculosis (combined 3.0 million), alcohol use (2.3 million), child and maternal malnutrition (1.4 million) and road accidents (1.4 million) are less potent. Moreover, inhaled PM accounts for ca. eight times as many deaths as drug use or all causes of violence (ca. 0.6 million). Only noncommunicable diseases such as dietary risk factors (all combined; 12.1 million) and hypertension (10.7 million) caused more deaths than (all types of) pollution.

On a geographical scale, most of the PM-related death toll normalized to population density is currently observed in African and Asian countries with more than 1,000 DALY per 100,000 people, but also in eastern Europe albeit with less than 1,000 DALY and to an even lesser degree in central European countries (Figure 10.6). On the other hand, northern America as well as Brazil, northern Africa, northern Europe and Australia are among the least affected countries with DALY of less than 679.

As stated above, in spite of the clear associations between PM concentration and health risks, epidemiologically derived associations should not be mistaken for causal links. Thus, corroborating evidence from other types of studies is required to confirm true causality between inhaled PM and health effects.

10.3.2 *Evidence from Clinical Studies*

To investigate the causes and relationships between exposure to inhaled aerosol and disease, several clinical studies have been conducted. In these studies, typically health volunteers and mildly diseases patients are exposed to low levels of inhaled particles under controlled conditions and a wide array of biomarkers is reported over a certain time period before, during and/or after the exposure. For ethical reasons, these studies were typically performed with healthy or mildly diseased volunteers at low exposure conditions, i.e., low-to-medium level PM concentration inhaled over a short period of time (typically a few hours). It is evident that under these conditions, only low levels of acute response parameters can be studied, no life-threatening chronic effects can be addressed. Moreover, the health effect estimates are likely too low, as they are not based on the most vulnerable parts of the population, namely elderly or already severely diseased patients. Most studies were conducted with carbonaceous particles resembling soot-dominated urban aerosol exposures. In spite of these limitations, clinical studies elucidate the biological response of humans to the inhalation of ambient PM albeit not for chronic long-term effects.

In the 2000s, a series of clinical inhalation studies was conducted at the University of Rochester, New York, USA, investigating the causal

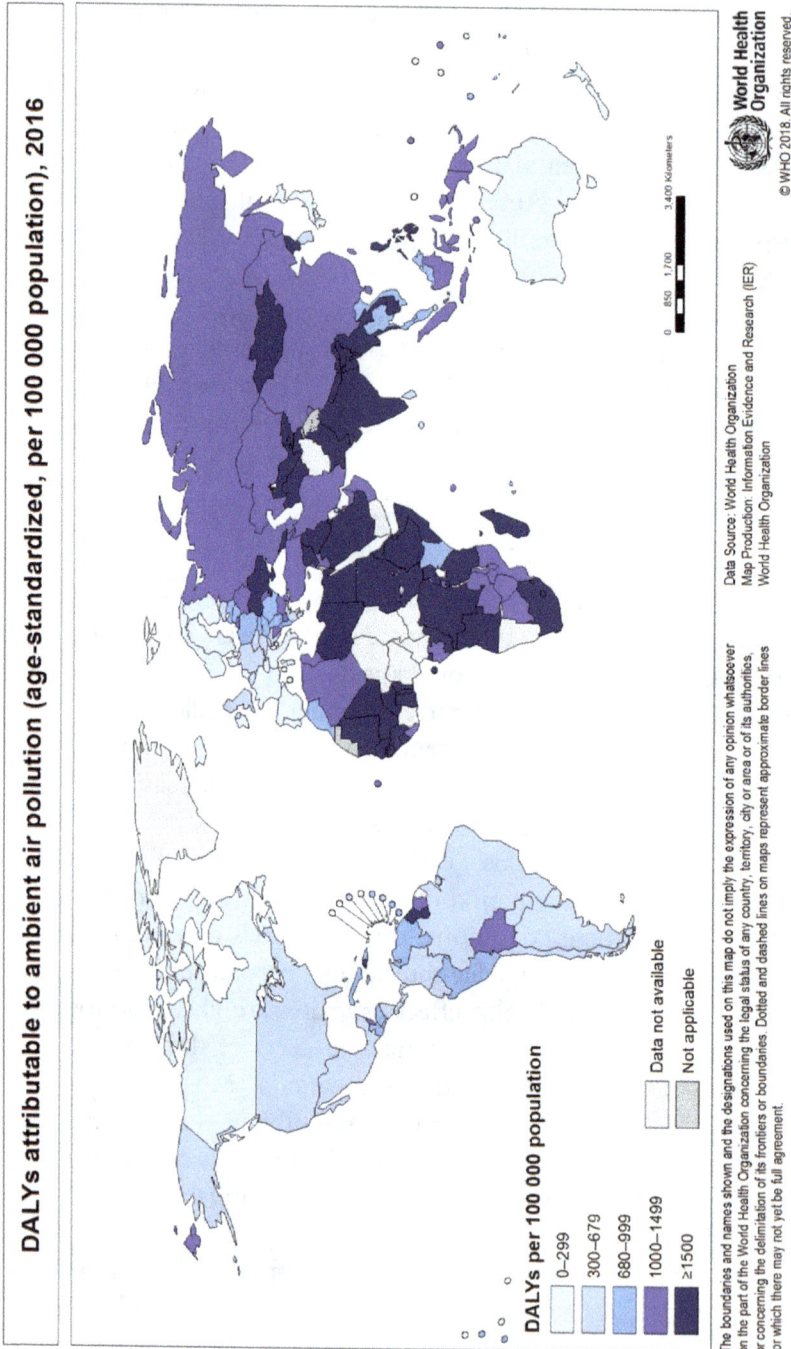

Figure 10.6: Disability-adjusted life years (DALY) lost per 100,000 people due to ambient air pollution (mainly PM inhalation) according to the records of the World Health Organization (WHO) from 2016.[6]

relationship between carbon particles and pulmonary and cardiovascular effects.[9] Healthy and potentially susceptible (mild-asthmatic) subjects were screened for various pulmonary and cardiovascular outcomes, including airway inflammation, blood coagulation and cardiac rhythm. The study was designed as a randomized, double-blind cross-over study, i.e., subjects inhaled either filtered air (control measurement) or carbon particles via a mouthpiece with a 2–3-week regeneration phase between two inhalations. A total of 56 subjects participated in the study (28 male, 28 female, age: 30 ± 10 years), with 40 healthy and 16 mild-asthma patients. The number and mass median diameter of the inhaled nanoparticle agglomerates was 25–35 nm and the nominal mass concentrations were 10, 25 and 50 $\mu g/m^3$ for healthy subjects and 10 $\mu g/m^3$ for low-asthmatic subjects corresponding to low- and medium-level urban concentrations by the standards of the western, industrialized world. The 2-h inhalations were carried out with or without moderate physical activity (healthy: 10, 25 and 50 $\mu g/m^3$, mild-asthmatic: 10 $\mu g/m^3$; cycling on ergometer) and rest periods in 15-min intervals alternated. Various biological parameters were observed at several time points up to 45 h after exposure.

These studies showed that in healthy volunteers with moderate physical activity only the highest concentration (50 $\mu g/m^3$) did induce a mild dysfunction in the small airways, coupled with a somewhat diminished alveolar gas exchange, but not in mild-asthmatic subjects at the highest investigated concentration (10 $\mu g/m^3$). Whether similar or perhaps more pronounced effects at 25 or 50 $\mu g/m^3$ would have been present in mild-asthmatic subjects could not be investigated in this study. Overall, no clear evidence of pulmonary or systemic inflammation was found in either healthy or mild-asthmatic volunteers. On the other hand, particle inhalation resulted in decreased maximum blood flow in the (hyperemic) upper arm, increased minimal blood vessel resistance, and decreased plasma nitrate levels. These results support the hypothesis that PM inhalation impairs vascular function and reduces the bioavailability of nitric oxide. Overall, most of the investigated response parameters showed no effect and only a few — mainly cardiovascular endpoints — showed a mild response to repeated short term inhalation of soot-like carbon particles.[10,11]

Another study showed that 2-h inhalation of soot-like carbon nanoparticles resulted in transient activation of blood platelets and possibly the vascular endothelium in type 2 diabetes patients. This could be an indication of an increased cardiovascular risk for type 2 diabetes patients associated with ambient PM inhalation, although no comparative study was conducted with healthy volunteers.[12]

In summary, numerous clinical studies on the effect of diesel soot (or soot-like) nanoparticles on health indicate that soot exposure can lead to short-term effects, especially with regard to pulmonary, cardiovascular and neurologic effects. This supports the PM-health associations reported by epidemiologic studies and provides evidence for causal links between PM inhalation and adverse health effects, albeit not for chronic effects after long-term exposure of the potentially most susceptible part of the population (elderly and severely diseased). However, it is not clear whether these effects are associated only with the particle components of diesel exhaust or if gas phase components also contribute.[13]

10.3.3 *Evidence from Toxicological Studies*

To close the knowledge gap on the health implications of high dose, long-term PM exposures, one has to resort to toxicological studies with model organisms — not humans. Numerous PM-related studies have been performed with both *in vitro* cell culture and *in vivo* animal models. Any of these model organisms cannot fully mimic the human health scenario, but typically one considers more complex organisms such as animals (often rodents like mice and rats) as more predictive for human health than *in vitro* cell culture models, albeit complex cell models as potential alternatives to animal testing are currently under development. Here, we present toxicological data from animal models.

One of the most important issues, which cannot be investigated easily in epidemiological and clinical studies, is the relevance of different dose metrics for the prediction of PM-induced health effects. Historically, mass has been the most widely used dose metric, but surface area, number and even volume have also been proposed as relevant dose metrics for biopersistent particles (i.e., particles that are not completely dissolved within a matter of days such as soot, but not sea salt or other biologically degradable materials). Figure 10.7 shows that surface area dose, but not mass or number shows a strong correlation with the observed neutrophil influx — a hallmark of pulmonary inflammation — into the lungs of mice and rats 24 h after pulmonary application of various doses of different types of biopersistent nano-sized particles (primary diameter below 300 nm). This is evident from the correlation coefficient R of near unity for surface area as dose metric ($R^2 = 0.78$, i.e., 78% of the observed variability in inflammation can be explained by changes in surface area dose), while considerably lower R^2 values (<0.5) are obtained for mass (or volume) and number as dose metric.[14] Similar results have been found for chronic health effects such as the induction of lung cancer in rats.[15] Early studies on the effect of particle size have often indicated that smaller particles (especially nano-sized particles with diameter <100 nm) are more toxic than micron-sized particles (>1 μm). However, this finding is mostly an artifact of using mass as dose metric, because smaller particles have a larger surface area per mass than larger particles.

The effect of particle size and even of chemical composition is largely eliminated, if surface area is used as dose metric (Figure 10.7, panel A). Thus, using surface area instead of mass as dose metric, combines many materials into one toxicity class, while this is not the case for mass as dose metric. The superiority of surface area over mass as dose metric for particle toxicity is intuitively clear, because for biopersistent materials, as considered here, only the surface area is in direct contact with the biological matrix. The interior of a particle does not directly interact with the biological matrix and is therefore not relevant for the toxicological particle effects. This finding is starting to impact regulatory bodies in their quest for the definition of safe limits of particle exposure. Using surface area as dose metric, one can group various transition metals into a class with elevated surface-specific toxicity (e.g., zinc-, copper-, nickel-oxide). These materials have an about 12-fold enhanced surface-specific toxicity as compared to the so-called low solubility, low toxicity (LSLT) materials presented in Figure 10.7 (panel

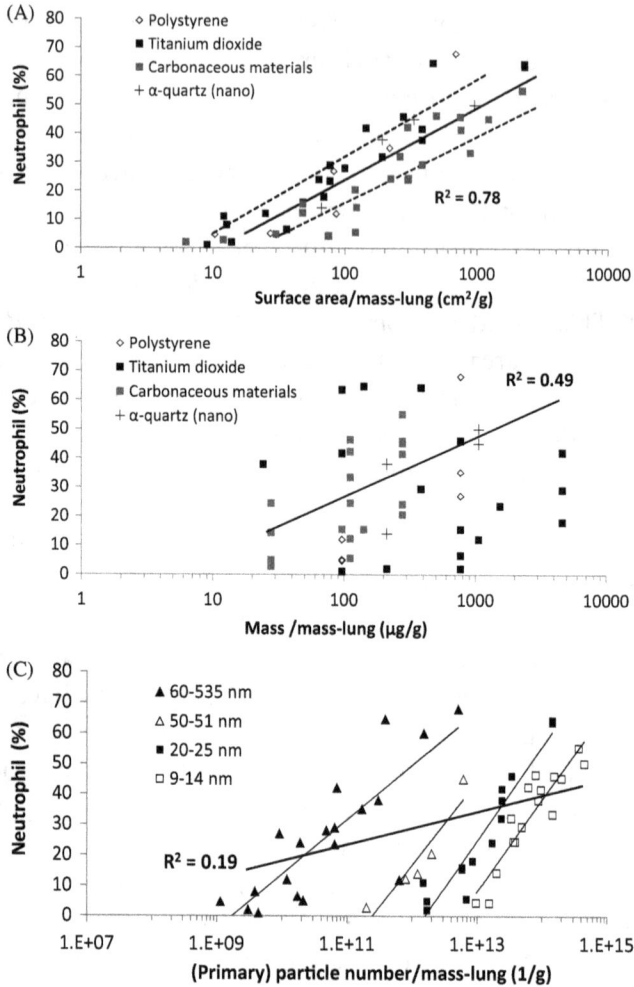

Figure 10.7:   Acute pulmonary inflammation as measured by neutrophil influx into the lungs of rats and mice 24 h after pulmonary application of nanoparticles of different chemical composition and (primary) particle diameter. Most of the carbonaceous materials refer to soot-like particles, one of the most common components in ambient urban PM. It is evident that surface area (normalized to lung weight) is the toxicologically most relevant dose metric, not mass or number (of primary particles) (Adapted from Ref. 14.).

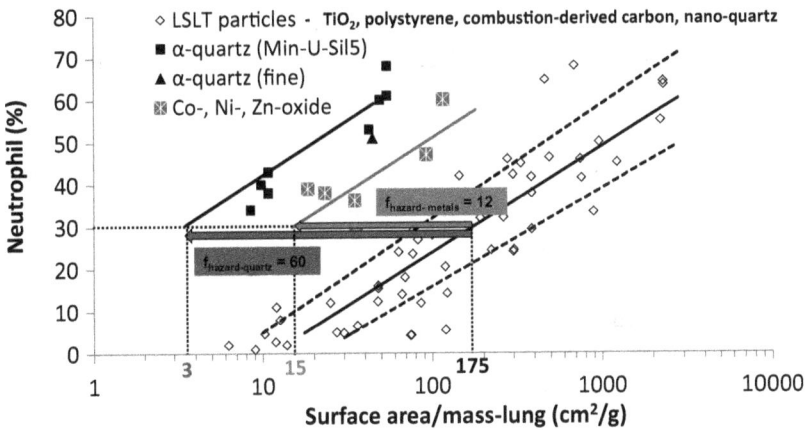

Figure 10.8: Same acute pulmonary inflammation data as presented in Figure 10.7 (panel A, open symbols) extended by data from α-crystalline quartz and various oxides of transition metals (copper-, nickel-, zinc-oxide) (Adapted from Ref. 14.).

A), as they reach the same level of (acute) pulmonary inflammation (here: 30% neutrophil influx) at a 12-fold lower dose (15 instead of 175 cm²/g) (Figure 10.8).[14] Crystalline quartz (SiO_2) is even more toxic; it has a 60-fold enhanced toxicity as compared to LSLT materials. These so-called hazard factors can be utilized to define occupational exposure limits for particles of different toxicity classes (see Chapter 12).

It is important to note that the carbonaceous materials included in Figure 10.7 closely resemble soot particles, which are considered one of the main contributors to the toxicity of ambient urban PM. Thus, it is likely that surface area is also the most relevant dose metric for urban PM, but this has not been confirmed by epidemiological studies mainly due to the lack of reliable surface area dose measurements at urban PM monitoring sites. As a surrogate for surface area, it has been shown that ambient particle number concentration can be a predictor of soot-dominated near-source health effects, but this is not always the case — probably because it is not particle number but surface area that is the most relevant dose metric.

Toxicological studies also offer an opportunity to study the types of adverse effects and the underlying mechanisms of disease induced by long-term, chronic PM exposure. In addition to pulmonary inflammation (both acute and chronic), lung cancer, cardiovascular effects and pulmonary fibrosis have been identified as main adverse outcomes (AOs). Moreover, immunomodulatory effects on inhaled PM have been demonstrated. At least an adjuvant role of PM exposure in the degree of allergy and asthma symptoms have been observed, and there are also indications that exposure to soot particles can activate dormant viruses, which could result in higher prevalence of infectious diseases.[16] Effects of PM exposure on other types of diseases such as neurodegenerative diseases or diabetes are currently under investigation. These toxicological findings are in general agreement with results from epidemiological studies as described above.[5,17,18]

For fiber- or tube-like particles — not included in Figure 10.7 — exceeding a certain length (>5 μm) and stiffness, there is evidence that it is not surface area but number, which is the more relevant dose metric. Upon particle deposition in the alveolar region of the lung, macrophages get activated to clear these particles by cellular internalization (phagocytosis). For particles larger than 5–10 μm, this process is inhibited, because it exceeds the dimensions of a macrophage. For fiber-like particles, this inhibition mechanism fails, because the diameter of fiber-like particles is much smaller than 5 μm, which allows initiation but not completion of phagocytosis, resulting in the destruction of the macrophage (frustrated phagocytosis). As this process is related to the number of fiber-like particles rather than their surface area, number is considered the toxicologically most relevant dose metric for long (>5 μm) fiber-like particles.[19]

For a reduction of the PM-induced health effects with attention to specific toxicity classes, an understanding of the biological mechanisms involved in disease development is required. Toxicological studies offer a unique opportunity of addressing this issue. Exposure studies with model organisms allow for dose-controlled exposures with different types of aerosol, while excluding confounding factors such as noise and exposure to other co-pollutants such as ozone. Moreover, temporal changes of the health/disease status of the organism can be monitored in the entire organism on all scales of

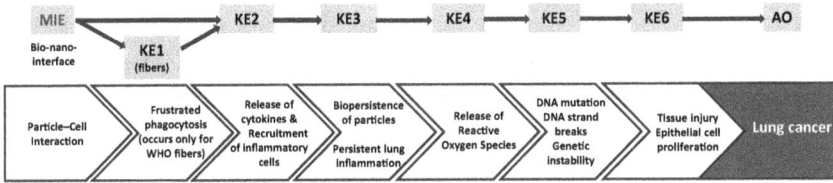

Figure 10.9: Example of an adverse outcome pathway (AOP) linking inhaled particles to lung cancer. The origin of each AOP is a molecular initiating event (MIE), which leads over one or more than one (here six) biological key events (KE) to an adverse outcome (AO). Each of these steps should be confirmed by experimental evidence and ultimately dose-response relations for each of these steps will allow the definition of safe exposure levels.

interest including genetic response, changes in cell signaling or protein secretion and physiological and structural changes in the organism. Often, genetic modification of an organism may allow for deactivation and/or activation of specific genes, which is an important tool to identify causal links between genetic profiles and disease development. Ultimately, toxicological risk assessment of any chemical substance such as inhaled particles requires the definition of a so-called adverse outcome pathway (AOP). The AOP links in a linear way existing knowledge along a series of causally connected *key events* (KE) between two points — a *molecular initiating event* (MIE) and an AO that occur at a level of biological organization relevant to risk assessment. As an example, Figure 10.9 provides one version of the currently discussed AOP for PM-induced cancer due to fiber-like and spherical (KE1 not included) particles. The classification of particles based on AOP and associated hazard factors (see Figure 10.8) are becoming increasingly more important for expanding the use of mechanistic toxicological data to risk assessment and regulatory measures of exposure control (Chapter 12).

10.4 Conclusion

The combined evidence from epidemiological, clinical and toxicological studies indicates that exposure to inhaled PM, which is biopersistent in biological matrices (e.g., soot), enhances the risk of morbidity and mortality mainly due to cardiovascular and pulmonary effects. A thorough understanding of the AOP is essential for PM-related risk assessment and regulatory measures. The burden of disease and premature death induced by PM inhalation is similar, albeit somewhat lower, to that of cigarette smoking. Lung-deposited surface area dose is the most relevant dose metric for biopersistent PM. However, due to the current lack of reliable and standardized methods for surface area monitoring, mass and number measurements will remain important for regulatory purposes. Finally, the toxicologically derived dose-response curves can only be related to epidemiological exposure levels, if the inhaled aerosol concentration is converted into equivalent lung-deposited dose. Fundamental knowledge of aerosol science as described here is essential for this.

References

1. Landrigan PJ, Fuller R, Acosta NJR, Adeyi O, Arnold R, Basu N, Balde AB, Bertollini R, Bose-O'Reilly S, Boufford JI, Breysse PN, Chiles T, Mahidol C, Coll-Seck AM, Cropper ML, Fobil J, Fuster V, Greenstone M, Haines A, Hanrahan D, Hunter D, Khare M, Krupnick A, Lanphear B, Lohani B, Martin K, Mathiasen KV, McTeer MA, Murray CJL, Ndahimananjara JD, Perera F, Potocnik J, Preker AS, Ramesh J, Rockstrom J, Salinas C, Samson LD, Sandilya K, Sly PD, Smith KR, Steiner A, Stewart RB, Suk WA, van Schayck OCP, Yadama GN, Yumkella K, and Zhong M. (2018). The Lancet Commission on pollution and health. *Lancet* **391**: 462–512.
2. ICRP. (1994). International Commission on Radiological Protection (ICRP), Human respiratory tract model for radiological protection: A report of a task group of the ICRP. In: *ICRP Publication 66; Annals of the ICRP*. Oxford, UK: Elsevier Science Ltd., pp. 1–482.
3. Pope CA. (1996). Particulate pollution and health: A review of the Utah valley experience. *J. Expo. Anal. Environ. Epidemiol.* **6**: 23–34.
4. Schleicher N, Norra S, Chen YZ, Chai FH, and Wang SL. (2012). Efficiency of mitigation measures to reduce particulate air pollution — A case study during the Olympic Summer Games 2008 in Beijing, China. *Sci. Total Environ.* **427**: 146–158.
5. Peters A, Ruckerl R, and Cyrys J. (2011). Lessons from air pollution epidemiology for studies of engineered nanomaterials. *J. Occup. Environ. Med.* **53**: S8–S13.

6. WHO. (2016). Global Burden of Disease Study of World Health Organisation (WHO). https://www.who.int/gho/map_gallery/en/, **Accessed 11 June 2019**.

7. COMEAP. (2010). The Mortality Effects of Long-Term Exposure to Particulate Air Pollution in the United Kingdom, Committee on the Medical Effects of Air Pollutants (COMEAP). http://www.comeap.org.uk/subgroups/51-the-mortality-effects-of-long-term-exposure-to-particulate-air-pollution-in-the-united-kingdom, **Accessed 15 July 2013**.

8. Pope CA, Ezzati M, and Dockery DW. (2009). Fine-particulate air pollution and life expectancy in the United States. *N. Eng. J. Med.* **360**: 376–386.

9. Frampton MW, Utell MJ, Zareba W, Oberdörster G, Cox C, Huang LS, Morrow PE, Lee FE, Chalupa D, Frasier LM, Speers DM, and Stewart J. (2004). Effects of exposure to ultrafine carbon particles in healthy subjects and subjects with asthma. *Res. Rep. Health Eff. Inst.* 1–47; discussion 49–63.

10. Shah AP, Pietropaoli AA, Frasier LM, Speers DM, Chalupa DC, Delehanty JM, Huang LS, Utell MJ, and Frampton MW. (2008). Effect of inhaled carbon ultrafine particles on reactive hyperemia in healthy human subjects. *Environ. Health Perspect.* **116**: 375–380.

11. Pietropaoli AP, Frampton MW, Hyde RW, Morrow PE, Oberdörster G, Cox C, Speers DM, Frasier LM, Chalupa DC, Huang LS, and Utell MJ. (2004). Pulmonary function, diffusing capacity, and inflammation in healthy and asthmatic subjects exposed to ultrafine particles. *Inhal. Toxicol.* **16 Suppl 1**: 59–72.

12. Zareba W, Couderc JP, Oberdorster G, Chalupa D, Cox C, Huang LS, Peters A, Utell MJ, and Frampton MW. (2009). ECG parameters and exposure to carbon ultrafine particles in young healthy subjects. *Inhal. Toxicol.* **21**: 223–233.

13. Hesterberg TW, Long CM, Lapin CA, Hamade AK, and Valberg PA. (2010). Diesel exhaust particulate (DEP) and nanoparticle exposures: What do DEP human clinical studies tell us about potential human health hazards of nanoparticles? *Inhal. Toxicol.* **22**: 679–694.

14. Schmid O, and Stoeger T. (2016). Surface area is the biologically most effective dose metric for acute nanoparticle toxicity in the lung. *J. Aerosol. Sci.* **99**: 133–143.

15. Maynard AD, and Kuempel ED. (2005). Airborne nanostructured particles and occupational health. *J. Nanopart Res.* **7**: 587–614.

16. Sattler C, Moritz F, Chen S, Steer B, Kutschke D, Irmler M, Beckers J, Eickelberg O, Schmitt-Kopplin P, Adler H, and Stoeger T. (2017).

Nanoparticle exposure reactivates latent herpesvirus and restores a signature of acute infection. *Part Fibre Toxicol.* **14**: 2.

17. Schulz H, Harder V, Ibald-Mulli A, Khangdoga A, Koenig GW, Krombach F, Radykewicz R, Stampfl A, Thorand B, and Peters A. (2005). Cardiovascular effects of fine and ultrafine particles. *J. Aerosol Med.* **18**: 1–22.

18. Oberdörster G, Oberdörster E, and Oberdörster J. (2005). Nanotoxicology: An emerging discipline evolving from studies of ultrafine particles. *Environ. Health Perspect.* **113**: 823–839.

19. Shvedova AA, Yanamala N, Kisin ER, Tkach AV, Murray AR, Hubbs A, Chirila MM, Keohavong P, Sycheva LP, Kagan VE, and Castranova V. (2014). Long-term effects of carbon containing engineered nanomaterials and asbestos in the lung: One year postexposure comparisons. *Am. J. Physiol. Lung. Cell Mol. Physiol.* **306**: L170–L182.

Chapter 11
Aerosols in Unusual Environments

Chapter 9 describes situations in which there is inadvertent or occupational exposure to inhaled aerosols, and Chapter 10 details some of the adverse health consequences of such exposures. Such exposures are important in the context of environmental and occupational exposure because they can involve very large numbers of people, and thus they have important implications in matters pertaining to public health.

In contrast, this chapter discusses unusual situations to which few people will likely be exposed, but which serve to illustrate some of the points raised in previous chapters.

11.1 Altered Gravity

A large proportion of the inhaled particles that enter our lungs fall within the size range of ~8 – ~0.5 μm in size, and for those particles, the dominant mechanism of deposition is gravitational sedimentation (see Chapter 3 for details). As a direct consequence, a change in the g-level (be it an increase or a decrease) would be expected to alter aerosol transport and deposition in the lung.

Altered gravity environments are almost never seen on the Earth. Indeed, for all of evolution, gravity has remained essentially constant providing an acceleration towards the center of the Earth of 9.81 m/s², or 1G. It is only possible to alter the apparent force of gravity for those of us confined to the planet using high-speed aircraft or rotating centrifuges. Such environments are at best transient in nature, typically providing (apparent) altered gravity for periods of seconds to maybe minutes. For the very few of us that venture to space, micro-gravity (μG; zero-g, free-fall) can be experienced for sustained periods of time. In the future, planetary exploration may result in sustained periods of time spent in gravitation fields less than 1G, although the likelihood of long periods in sustained hypergravity seems remote given the distances involved in reaching planets with a mass larger than that of the Earth.

11.1.1 *Microgravity*

In terms of human exposure, μG periods of durations that are suffi-ciently long to make a meaningful measurement only occur during parabolic aircraft flight, or in spaceflight. In parabolic flight, the air-craft flies a maneuver, not unlike the trajectory of a roller coaster, and as the aircraft moves from a nose-high to a nose-low attitude, occu-pants are exposed to a period of free-fall or μG in the cabin for periods of up to ~25 s.[1] Although short-lived, these periods provide enough time to make some meaningful measurements and two of us (CD and GKP) have made extensive use of this in elucidating the role of gravity on aerosol transport and deposition.

11.1.1.1 *Aerosol deposition*

The first studies of aerosol deposition changes in μG used 2 μm monodisperse particles and a tyndallometer to measure particle con-centration in the airstream.[2] They showed an essentially linear increase in the deposition as a function of gravity level. As expected, there was still some deposition of particles in μG because although gravitational sedimentation was absent, other nongravitational deposition mecha-nisms were still active (Figure 11.1). Later studies[3] showed the same linear increase in deposition with increasing gravity for 2 and 3 μm particles (Figure 11.1), but notably for smaller particles (0.5 and 1 μm), deposition in μG was higher than expected, both in terms of maintaining a linear relationship with respect to gravity, and com-pared to the existing models of deposition. For the 0.5 and 1.0 μm

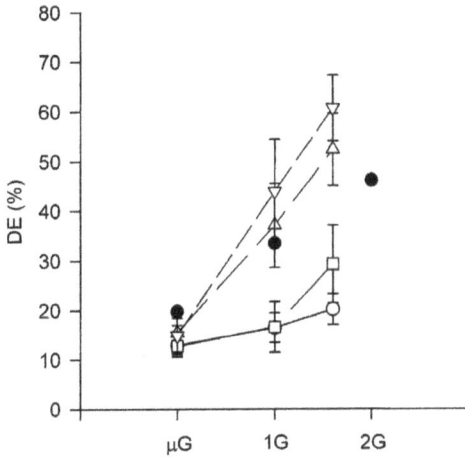

Figure 11.1: Total deposition in different gravity levels and with different sized particles (3 [downward triangle], 2 [upward triangle], 1 [open square] and 0.5 [open circle] μm). Results from the first-ever study of aerosol deposition in the human lung in microgravity (μG)[2] are superimposed and shown in the closed black circles. Note that for the 1 μm particles, deposition in μG is much higher than what would be suggested by the 1G and 2G data if one were to assume a linear function with respect to gravity (Used with permission from Ref. 3.)

particles, the deposition was approximately twice what was expected, suggesting some unaccounted for "enhanced diffusion" was operative, and that performing the studies in μG, where sedimentation was absent, unmasked this effect. Despite some subsequent studies,[4,5] a convincing explanation of the higher than anticipated deposition for small particles remained elusive.

In order for deposition to occur in the lung periphery, the inhaled particles must move from the inspired flow streamlines to the resident air in the lung. The particles that showed the greatest deviation from expectations in μG were those 1 μm in diameter, and diffusion distance for these particles in air is only ~13 μm, too short for diffusion to be effective at moving the particles. The most likely explanation for the unexpectedly high deposition is the concept of complex folding of the flow streamlines in the lung periphery.[6] This process is rather like the repeated stretching and folding of a sheet of pastry. The net effect is to bring points on the pastry sheet that were remote from each other into close apposition after folding. The complicated alveolar geometry means that a flow streamline during expiration experiences a different geometry to that which it experienced on inspiration. This non-reversibility of convective flow folds the streamlines around each other, bringing previously widely separated streamlines into close proximity, and in doing so, serves to provide an environment for the "enhanced diffusion" seen in μG deposition. Experimental attempts to demonstrate this effect, by imposing flow reversals during a breath-hold, suggested that the effect was already present in a single breath, although a definitive answer remains elusive.[7]

Bolus deposition studies (see Chapter 5) allow the probing of deposition at different points in the bronchial tree and provide useful insight into the overall process of deposition in reduced gravity. As would be expected by the removal of gravitational sedimentation, deposition is lower in reduced gravity than in 1G; however, the deposition that does occur is much more peripheral in the lung than in 1G. Specifically, a particular deposition level is reached at a greater penetration volume in reduced gravity than in normal gravity, suggesting that relative deposition in the lung periphery is increased in reduced gravity (Figure 11.2). In essence, it seems that gravity (i.e., sedimentation)

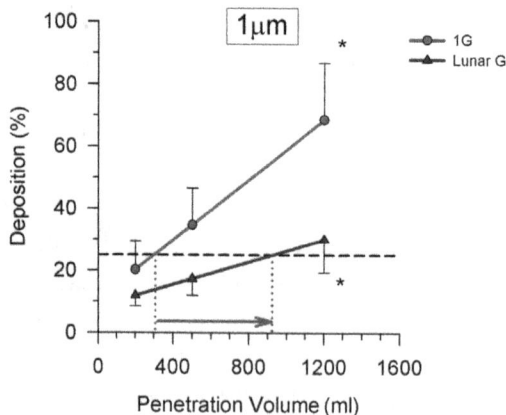

Figure 11.2: Bolus deposition of 1 μm particles in 1G and in Lunar gravity (1/6G) plotted as a function of the bolus penetration volume. Reduced gravity serves to reduce overall deposition, but those particles that are deposited do so in more peripheral lung regions as indicated by the red arrow (Redrawn and modified from Ref. 8.)

serves to effectively screen many particles from reaching the periphery of the lung. This effect has potential importance in the context of planetary exploration (see below) as particles that deposit peripherally are cleared more slowly than those deposited centrally (see Chapter 6), raising their potential for a toxicological insult.

11.1.1.2 *Aerosol clearance*

There is essentially no information on the rate of clearance of deposited aerosols in μG. Given the time constants associated with even the most rapid aspects of mucociliary clearance in the trachea (at least on the order of multiple minutes), parabolic flight does not provide a useful platform for such studies. There is a thought that useful measurements might be possible in the few minutes of μG that would be available in suborbital flight (essentially a huge parabolic maneuver), but such flights are not yet available. Clearance measurements would therefore require studies in orbital spaceflight, but the question of a suitable tracer remains unclear (short half-life tracers like ^{99m}Tc with a half-life of ~6 h cannot be used because of long delivery times to orbit), plus the challenges of flying radioactive materials are huge.

There are measurements that suggest a gravitational influence on mucociliary clearance velocity in the trachea of the horse as its gravitational orientation is altered.[9] However, the ability to translate these results to humans in μG is tenuous at best.

As there are no direct measurements of clearance rates in μG, we can only infer the residence time based on their site of deposition in the lung. As the amount of aerosol deposition is influenced by particles size (see Figure 11.1), it seems plausible that size will also have an effect on the site of deposition within the bronchial tree, with smaller particles able to penetrate more deeply into the lung periphery than large particles. This is certainly the case for terrestrial studies with smaller particles, depositing much more peripherally than coarse aerosols.[10]

Studies in reduced gravity that address the site of particle deposition are scarce. One such study in humans exposed to coarse (5 μm) ^{99m}Tc-labeled, delivered during μG, compared the pattern of

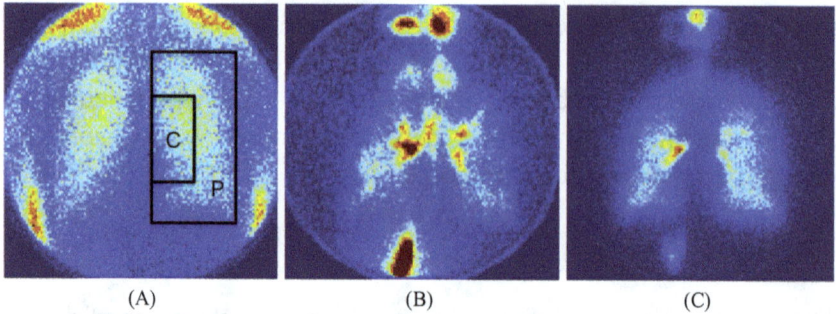

(A)   (B)   (C)

Figure 11.3: (A) Pattern of deposition of coarse (~5 µm) particles in microgravity (µG) and 1G. As expected, deposition was greatly reduced in µG compared to 1G; however, the central-to-peripheral deposition ratio indicates more peripheral deposition site in 1G due to the effects of gravitational sedimentation in 1G in the periphery. (A) is a transmission scan from a [57]Co planar source used to define the region of interest (outer black box) and the central and peripheral subregions (boxes labeled C and P, respectively). (B) The pattern of deposition of 5 µm particles labeled with ^{99m}Tc when the deposition occurred in (µG. (C) The pattern of deposition in the same subject when the deposition occurred in 1G (Used with permission from Ref. 11.)

deposition measured by planar gamma scintigraphy to that seen when the deposition occurred in 1G. To deposit an adequate dose, the tracer was administered over the course of several periods of µG during parabolic flights (Figure 11.3). The retention and distribution of deposited particles in the large, intermediate and small airways, and in the alveolar region, were determined through whole lung retention measurements (these were necessarily measured in 1G) post-inhalation and up to 22 h post-deposition (Figure 11.4). Somewhat counter to original expectations, the absence of gravitational sedimentation in µG caused relatively more particles to deposit in the larger (central) airways as a direct result of a decrease in peripheral deposition when sedimentation was eliminated, with alveolar deposition being only 17% of total deposition in µG, compared to ~58% for particles deposited in 1G. However, the overall deposition in µG was reduced, compared to that in 1G as expected.[11]

However, it seems that for fine particles (~1 µm), the situation is different. Unfortunately, there have not been any studies in humans on the actual site of deposition of fine particles in altered gravity levels. Some insight may however be gained from deposition of 1 µm

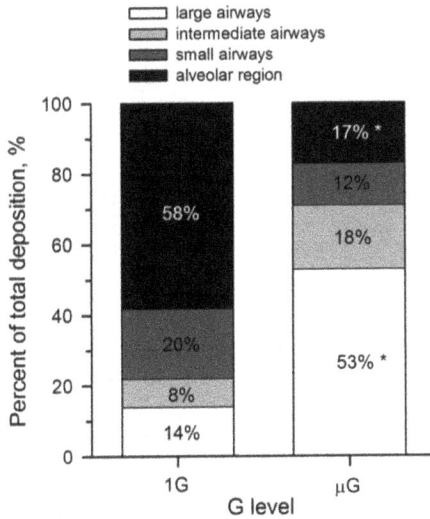

Figure 11.4: Estimates of the site of relative deposition in humans in μG and in 1G for coarse (~5 μm) particles (Used with permission from Ref. 11.)

ferromagnetic particles in rats in which the exposure occurred in μG and for which the deposition pattern was measured postmortem using magnetic resonance imaging of the excised and fixed lungs.[12,13] As was the case with the deposition of coarse particles, the total deposition was reduced in μG compared to that in 1G; however, for fine particles, the central-to-peripheral deposition ratio was reduced when deposition occurred in μG (see Figure 11.5). These data are consistent with an increase in the relative contribution of peripheral deposition to overall deposition and also with the inferential bolus measurements seen in Figure 11.2.

In the context of planetary exploration, the implication of these studies is that at least for the fine particle fraction, there may well be an increased residence time when the particles are deposited in low gravity, potentially raising their toxicological potential (see Section 11.2).

11.1.2 *Hypergravity*

As with μG, there are no habitats on the Earth that provide sustained hypergravity exposure for humans, although, in contrast to μG, such

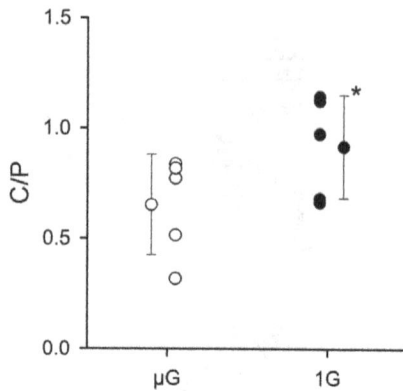

Figure 11.5:   Central-to-peripheral ratio of deposition if ~1 μm ferromagnetic particles in the lungs of rats measured either in μG or in 1G. Although absolute deposition in μG was reduced, relative deposition occurred more peripherally than in 1G as indicated by the C/P ratio (Used with permission from Ref. 13.)

habitats are at least theoretically possible. To our knowledge, there have been no studies on aerosol behavior in humans in sustained hypergravity.

However, during parabolic flight, the necessity to rapidly raise the nose of the aircraft prior to the zero-g portion of flight, and again following the zero-g period (when the aircraft is in a steep dive towards the ground!) provides short periods of hypergravity. In the US parabolic flight program, it is usual to fly a series of parabolas without a 1G pause between them, and so the period of hypergravity following the parabola and that which precedes the next parabola merge into one continuous hypergravity period. Although the aircraft maneuvering typically results in some variation in g-level (between ~1.2 and 1.8G), it is a reasonable approximation to consider this a period of 1.6G lasting ~45 s. To our knowledge, the only data on aerosol deposition in hypergravity in humans were collected by two of us (CD and GKP) in these short periods of hypergravity.

The effects are largely as expected, as illustrated in Figure 11.1, namely that as G level increases, so too does total deposition. As sedimentation is a linear function of gravity level, this is not particularly surprising, and the results are consistent with the numerical models of deposition.[3]

11.2 Aerosols and Planetary Exploration

Looking into the future, it seems plausible that humans will one day visit and likely live for extended periods of time on extra-terrestrial bodies. When that happens, a consideration of aerosol deposition and its consequences will be necessary. This section briefly addresses those factors.

11.2.1 *Effect of Altered Gas Composition/Density*

Currently, the International Space Station (ISS) maintains an internal atmosphere similar to that on the Earth at sea level (~760 mmHg, 21% O_2, albeit with a slightly elevated CO_2 of ~0.3–0.4%). However, this choice of atmosphere, while closely mimicking that on Earth, brings with it operational difficulties associated with extra-vehicular activity (EVA, Spacewalk) because the internal pressure in the space-suits is very low (~220 mmHg in the US suit, ~290 mmHg in the Russian suit, both using 100% O_2 to avoid hypoxia). This low pressure is required for suit mobility and the engineering challenges of making a practical high-pressure suit are formidable. However, the large reduction in absolute pressure coupled with the high (~79%) N_2 concentration in ISS means that the transition from ISS to the suit without first washing out dissolved N_2 from the body tissues would result in severe (and likely fatal) decompression sickness (the Bends). To avoid this, a complicated and lengthy denitrogenation protocol is used as the lead up to each EVA, and this requires ~4 h to complete, a significant mission overhead.

For this reason, when extraterrestrial habitats for planetary exploration are developed, it is unlikely that the atmosphere in them will mimic that on Earth. Instead, the likely atmosphere of a Lunar habitat is currently set at ~380 mmHg (half that at sea level) with an O_2 concentration of ~32%. This atmosphere is a compromise point between the need to reduce denitrogenation time by lowering the partial pressure of N_2 (through lowering absolute pressure), avoiding extreme hypoxia that might be deleterious to health (through raising the O_2 concentration), all the while avoiding an excessive fire risk that results from very high O_2 fractions in the atmosphere. This atmosphere reduces the required denitrogenation time to ~15 min without the need to use high-pressure suits. However, because the absolute pressure is low, so too is the gas density, and this has the potential to affect aerosol transport in the lung.

The combined effect of μG and lowered gas density was studied in parabolic flight.[14] It was not possible to lower the absolute pressure as would be the case in a Lunar habitat, and so the effects of reduced density were mimicked by breathing a gas containing helium to lower average density. To account for the difference in absolute pressure between the aircraft cabin and the ground, the helium concentration was tailored so that density was the same in both environments. The studies used μG and 1G as the two gravity conditions, with the reasoning that the maximum difference (if any) would be seen, and deposition in either Lunar (1/6G) or Martian (3/8G) gravity would be intermediate.

Reduced gravity had a large effect on deposition, but the effect of lowered gas density was comparatively small (Figure 11.6). The effect

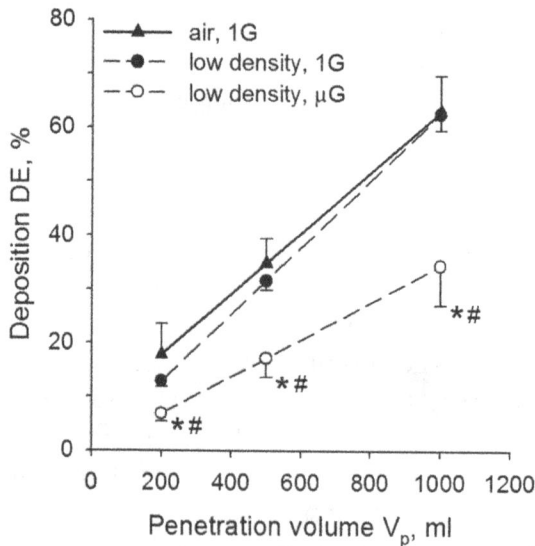

Figure 11.6: Aerosol bolus deposition of 1 μm particles when both gas density and gravity are altered. While gas density has a small but measurable effect on deposition at low bolus penetration volumes, gravity is a much more influential modulator (Used with permission from Ref. 14.)

seen was greatest at shallow penetration volumes (~200 mL), when reduced gas density served to lower deposition by ~23%. However, reduced gravity alone lowered deposition by ~47% and the combination of reduced density and reduced gravity lowered deposition by 59%. At deeper penetration volumes, the effect was smaller, which is consistent with the reduction in turbulent flow afforded by the lower density gas in the upper airways. The results suggest that the overall influence of a hypobaric habitat environment (which would serve to reduce gas density) is small compared to the influence of the reduced gravity that would be present in a Lunar or Martian habitat.

11.2.2 *Lunar Dust Toxicity*

The Apollo Lunar landing missions in 1969–1972 brought back ~484 kg of Lunar rocks, soil, and dust, and so there is a great deal known about the properties of Lunar dust (the most relevant component in terms of aerosol deposition). Of particular note is that ~10% of the lunar surface material is in the form of dust in the respirable range (<10 μm). While Lunar explorers will be protected from dust exposure by their spacesuits while outside on the Lunar surface, the Apollo experience showed that the dust tended to stick to the spacesuits was difficult to remove, and as a result, was tracked inside to the interior of the Lunar Module, so that the astronauts were exposed to the dust once their helmets were removed. Indeed, every Apollo mission debrief included comments from the crew about the dust, and how pervasive it was, and the LM pilot of Apollo 17 described an acrid smell from the dust as soon as he removed his helmet "as if a gun had been fired inside the cabin" (personal communication). Thus, the problem of dust is considered by NASA and ESA to be important in the context of Lunar and planetary exploration.

The toxicological properties of Lunar dust have been studied, mostly using so-called Lunar dust simulants, the most common being JSC-1A, a dust mixture made primarily from ash deposits from the San Francisco volcano in Arizona. Studies using both simulant and actual Lunar dust samples have explored their toxicity in rats using both intratracheal instillation and inhalation of aerosolized dust.

A nose-only inhalation study exposed rats to ground Lunar dust with a particles size of ~2 µm, and used comparably sized quartz and TiO_2 as the positive and negative controls, respectively.[15] The results were largely comparable to prior studies using Lunar dust simulant[16,17] and showed the toxicity, assessed by numerous end-points to be intermediate to the controls. The key outcome was setting a permissible exposure level (PEL) of between 0.5 and 1.0 mg/m³ for periodic exposures during a stay in a Lunar habitat.[18] NASA has subsequently implemented a more conservative PEL of 0.3 mg/m³.

A potentially important difference exists between the JSC-1A simulant and actual Lunar dust in that the latter is known to include encapsulated particles of iron in the zero valence state (Fe^0), a state not found on Earth due to oxidative processes that are absent on the Lunar surface (the Moon has no atmosphere). Evidence from chemical studies suggests that this so-called nano-phase iron may increase the reactivity of the dust,[19] although this has not been borne out in the limited toxicity studies performed to date.

The lack of any atmosphere on the Lunar surface has itself implications in terms of the toxicity of the dust. The mechanism by which Lunar dust is generated is a meteoric bombardment of the Lunar surface, and this results in shock melting of the impacted rock and subsequent agglomeration of particles. As a result, many of the lunar dust particles have high surface area to volume ratios, and as surface area is important in toxicity potential, this may be an important aspect to consider.[20]

The other consequence of the lack of a Lunar atmosphere is that there is no means by which the fractured particles resulting from meteoric impact can have any surface reactivity decreased by oxidative processes. Thus, although the fracturing of the dust grain surface may have happened millennia ago, the dust is in effect "fresh-fractured," As fresh-fractured crystalline quartz is known to have a high toxicological potential, the same may be true of Lunar dust on the Lunar surface. This may also account for the observation regarding the smell of the dust observed in Apollo 17. Further, the radiation environment on the lunar surface both from solar particles and galactic cosmic rays/ions may serve to promote surface reactivity. However, virtually all of the

Lunar dust samples that were returned by the Apollo missions were stored under a pure nitrogen atmosphere and while this is thought to have slowed oxidation, it did not eliminate it. Some samples were sealed on the Lunar surface under vacuum conditions, but to date, these few samples have never been opened and it is therefore unknown if the vacuum has been maintained in these special sample canisters, nor if the surface reactivity of these samples is higher than Lunar dust stored under N_2. Studies of freshly ground samples of coarse Lunar dust (ground under vacuum) have suggested increased chemical reactivity but there have been no toxicity studies performed with such material. At least one study has shown that the time required for a reduction in the surface activity of quartz dust to half its original level following grinding is on the order of 4 h. This suggests that exposure to Lunar dust that has been tracked into an airlock and that might be inhaled during removal of a space suit may have a much greater toxicological potential that the "passivated" dust used in the rat studies described above. It seems likely that any questions surrounding the surface reactivity of Lunar dust will have to await a future Lunar sample return mission, which includes an appropriately stored dust sample.

11.2.3 *Martian Dust*

A limited amount is known about Martian dust, as there have been no sample return missions from Mars. However, unlike the Moon, Mars has an atmosphere (albeit a rather thin one) and so chemical weathering of the dust present almost certainly occurs. There have been a number of Martian lander missions that have included in situ chemical analyses and these have shown high iron content in Martian soils primarily in the Fe^{3+} oxidative state (the same as terrestrial rust), hence the red color of Mars. Some Martian meteorites are found on Earth and these provide a very limited window into the nature of Martian dust. However, Mars routinely experiences dust storms, which, given the thin atmosphere, suggest a considerable degree of fine particles. While the possibly highly oxidative nature of Lunar dust may not be an issue on Mars, the presence and effects of dust will likely present significant mission impacts for exploration missions.

Martian dust is also known to contain a perchlorate component as well as a hexavalent chromium component, although data to date suggest that these are sufficiently small to not be of great concern.[22]

11.2.4 *Asteroids*

The other possibility for extra-terrestrial exploration is that of near-Earth objects (NEOs), which typically means asteroids and comets. As is the case with Mars, there have been no sample return missions, but observations from probes such as Rosetta show dusty surfaces, which, given the lack of atmosphere, suggests that asteroid dust may be similar to Lunar dust, although the same may not be the case for comets that contain significant amounts of water. However, as with the Moon and Mars, dust will need to be a consideration in any explorations of NEOs.

References

1. Karmali F, and Shelhamer M. (2008). The dynamics of parabolic flight: Flight characteristics and passenger percepts. *Acta. Astronaut.* **63**: 594–602.
2. Hoffman RA, and Billingham J. (1975). Effect of altered G levels on deposition of particulates in the human respiratory tract. *J. Appl. Physiol.* **38**: 955–960.
3. Darquenne C, Paiva M, West JB, and Prisk GK. (1997). Effect of microgravity and hypergravity on deposition of 0.5- to 3-μm-diameter aerosol in the human lung. *J. Appl. Physiol.* **83**: 2029–2036.
4. Darquenne C, West JB, and Prisk GK. (1998). Deposition and dispersion of 1 μm aerosol boluses in the human lung: Effect of micro- and hypergravity. *J. Appl. Physiol.* **85**: 1252–1259.
5. Darquenne C, Paiva M, and Prisk GK. (2000). Effect of gravity on aerosol dispersion and deposition in the human lung after periods of breath-holding. *J. Appl. Physiol.* **89**: 1787–1792.
6. Tsuda A, Rogers RA, Hydon PE, and Butler JP. (2002). Chaotic mixing deep in the lung. *Proc. Natl. Acad. Sci. U. S. A.* **99**: 10173–10178.
7. Darquenne C, and Prisk GK. (2004). Effect of small flow reversals on aerosol mixing in the alveolar region of the human lung. *J. Appl. Physiol.* **97**: 2083–2089.

8. Darquenne C, and Prisk G. (2008). Deposition of inhaled particles in the human lung is more peripheral in lunar than in normal gravity. *Eur. J. Appl. Physiol.* **103**: 687–695.

9. Raidal S, Love D, and Bailey G. (1996). Effects of posture and accumulated airway secretions on tracheal mucociliary transport in the horse. *Aust. Vet. J.* **73**: 45–49.

10. Ilowite JS, Smaldone GC, Perry RJ, Bennett WD, and Foster WM. (1989). Relationship between tracheobronchial particle clearance rates and sites of initial deposition in man. *Arch. Environ. Health* **44**: 267–273.

11. Darquenne C, Zeman KL, Sa RC, Cooper TK, Fine JM, Bennett WD, and Prisk GK. (2013). Removal of sedimentation decreases relative deposition of coarse particles in the lung periphery. *J. Appl. Physiol.* **115**: 546–555.

12. Oakes JM, Scadeng M, Breen EC, Prisk GK, and Darquenne C. (2013). Regional distribution of aerosol deposition in rat lungs using magnetic resonance imaging. *Ann. Biomed. Eng.* **41**: 967–978.

13. Darquenne C, Borja MG, Oakes JM, Breen EC, Olfert IM, Scadeng M, and Prisk GK. (2014). Increase in relative deposition of fine particles in the rat lung periphery in the absence of gravity. *J. Appl. Physiol.* **117**: 880–886.

14. Darquenne C, and Prisk GK. (2013). Particulate deposition in the human lung under lunar habitat conditions. *Aviat. Space Environ. Med.* **84**: 190–195.

15. Lam CW, Scully RR, Zhang Y, Renne RA, Hunter RL, McCluskey RA, Chen BT, Castranova V, Driscoll KE, Gardner DE, McClellan RO, Cooper BL, McKay DS, Marshall L, and James JT. (2013). Toxicity of lunar dust assessed in inhalation-exposed rats. *Inhal. Toxicol.* **25**: 661–678.

16. Lam CW, James JT, Latch JN, Hamilton RF, Jr., and Holian A. (2002). Pulmonary toxicity of simulated lunar and Martian dusts in mice: II. Biomarkers of acute responses after intratracheal instillation. *Inhal. Toxicol.* **14**: 917–928.

17. Lam CW, James JT, McCluskey R, Cowper S, Balis J, and Muro-Cacho C. (2002). Pulmonary toxicity of simulated lunar and Martian dusts in mice: I. Histopathology 7 and 90 days after intratracheal instillation. *Inhal. Toxicol.* **14**: 901–916.

18. James JT, Lam CW, Santana PA, and Scully RR. (2013). Estimate of safe human exposure levels for lunar dust based on comparative benchmark dose modeling. *Inhal. Toxicol.* **25**: 243–256.

19. Wallace WT, Phillips CJ, Jeevarajan AYS, Chen B, and Taylor LA. (2010). Nano-phase iron-enhanced chemical reactivity of ground lunar soil. *Earth Planet. Sci. Lett.* **295**: 571–577.
20. Linnarsson D, Carpenter J, Fubini B, Gerde P, Karlsson LL, Loftus DJ, Prisk GK, Staufer U, Tranfield EM, and van Westrenen W. (2012). Toxicity of Lunar dust. *Planet. Space Sci.* **74**: 57–71.
21. Wallace WT, Taylor LA, Liu Y, Cooper BL, McKay DS, Chen B, and Jeevarajan AS. (2009). Lunar dust and lunar simulant activation and monitoring. *Meteoritics & Planetary Science* **44**: 961–970.
22. Levine JS, Winterhalter D, and Kerschmann RL. (2018). *Dust in the Atmosphere of Mars and its Impact on Human Exploration*. Cambridge, UK: Cambridge Scholars Publishing.

Chapter 12
Regulation of Particle Exposure

12.1 Introduction

Inhaled aerosols affect the health of more people than any other pollutant. They mainly originate from ambient aerosol sources, but indoor sources in private homes and occupational settings also play a significant role (Chapters 9 and 10). The most health-damaging particles or particulate matter (PM) are those with a diameter of 10 μm or less, (PM_{10}), which can penetrate and lodge deep inside the lungs. Chronic exposure to particles contributes to the risk of developing cardiovascular and respiratory diseases, as well as lung cancer and other diseases (Chapter 10). Consequently, regulatory measures have been taken to limit PM_{10}, $PM_{2.5}$ and/or $PM_{0.1}$ exposure to levels that are considered "safe" based on the available body of evidence.

Air quality measurements are typically reported in terms of daily or annual mean concentrations of particles. Routine air quality measurements typically describe such PM concentrations in terms of micrograms per cubic meter of air ($\mu g/m^3$). When sufficiently sensitive measurement tools are available, concentrations of fine particles ($PM_{2.5}$ or smaller), are also reported. It has been described above that airborne particles can only induce adverse health effects, if they come in contact with the lung (Chapter 10). Thus, it is not the PM concentration in air, but rather the lung-deposited dose expressed in terms of delivered particle mass (or surface area) per surface area of lung epithelium ($\mu g/cm^2$ or cm^2 — PM/cm^2 — lung) that is toxicologically the most relevant dose metric. Yet, because of the lack of

193

well-established measurement methods for lung-deposited dose or particle surface area concentration in air, regulatory particle exposure limits are currently based on particle mass concentrations ($\mu g/m^3$) in ambient air. The only exception is occupational exposure limits (OELs) for fiber-like particles, which are based on particle number concentration (particles/m^3 or $1/m^3$). In principle, there is a well-defined relationship between exposure concentration and lung-deposited particle dose, which depends on size distribution and chemical composition (hygroscopic growth) of the particles and respiratory conditions (Chapter 10). For many practical purposes, the use of average conditions is sufficient for relating particle concentration and dose. But the limitations of exposure concentration to predict pulmonary dose and health outcome need to be recognized to avoid inadvertent underestimation of health risks for specific exposure conditions such as specific occupational conditions.

12.2 Guidelines and Regulatory Limits of Particle Exposure

Decisions on legally binding exposure limits for particle exposure are made by regulatory bodies after a political process. This process is based on scientific recommendations (e.g., by the World Health Organization, WHO) and typically takes years, as it needs to balance conflicting interests such as protection of public health, economic stability and public welfare, including protection against decreased visibility, damage to animals, crops, vegetation and buildings. In light of the complexity of these socioeconomic conflicts, it is no surprise that different countries have adopted different exposure limits. These can apply over differing periods of time because the observed health effects associated with PM exposure occur on an acute (hours to days) to chronic time scale (months to lifetime).

12.2.1 *Ambient Air*

Table 12.1 provides an overview on current exposure limits for PM$_{2.5}$ in various countries — most of them are legally binding. None of these

Table 12.1: Guidelines and legally binding exposure limits for ambient $PM_{2.5}$[1]

Agency/country	Average limit ($\mu g/m^3$)		Comment	Year
	$PM_{2.5}$			
	Daily	Annual		
World Health Organization (WHO)	25	10	Legally non-binding Air Quality Guideline (mainly for developed countries)	2014
United States	35	12		2013
EU	—	25		2015
Australia	25	8	Established in 2003; not enforced until now	2003
Singapore	37.5	12		2015
Japan	35	15		2009
India	60	40		2009
China	35	15		2016

countries has implemented fully the guidelines recommended by the WHO for daily and annually averaged exposure levels of 25 and 10 $\mu g/m^3$, respectively, but all of the countries are converging toward these limits and do not exceed them by more than a factor of 2.5 and 4 for the daily and annual average exposure levels, respectively.

In contrast to $PM_{2.5}$, regulation of PM_{10} exposure is more difficult mainly due to the potentially large effect of natural sources such as deserts on ambient PM_{10} levels.

12.2.2 *Indoor Air — Private Home*

In addition to ambient PM exposure, indoor particle exposure can contribute substantially to the total PM burden. In private homes, PM sources and exposure levels are highly variable and strongly dependent on the country (Chapter 9). The most severe effect has been reported for low- and middle-income countries, where household fuel combustion and poor ventilation are among the most relevant and severe challenges for mitigation of indoor PM levels. In 2014, the WHO has introduced $PM_{2.5}$ guidelines for emission rates from household fuel combustion sources, which depend on the level of ventilation of the home[2]:

$$0.23 \ (\text{mg/min}) \ (\text{unvented})$$

$$0.80 \ (\text{mg/min}) \ (\text{vented})$$

However, these guidelines are just recommendations. To the best of our knowledge, there are currently no legally binding guidelines for PM exposure in private homes.

12.2.3 *Occupational Exposure Limits*

In the workplace, OELs for inhaled particles have been put into effect by regulatory bodies all over the world. Typically, OELs represent[3] 8-h mean PM concentration values at or below which adverse health effects do not appear in most workers working for 8 h a day, 40 h a week under a moderate work-load. Exposure concentrations above OEL should be avoided even for short durations or light work intensity. If mean levels and duration of exposure corresponding to segments of various jobs can be measured or estimated, then an overall exposure concentration can be determined as the time-weighted average concentration.

It is evident from Table 12.2 that the OELs vary considerably for different countries and exceed the ambient exposure limits by orders of magnitude. While the OEL for respirable nuisance dust, which has no specific toxicity such as quartz, some metal oxides or WHO fibers (long, thick fibers), ranges from 0.5 to 5 mg/m^3, the OEL corridor for quartz is relatively narrow (0.03–0.05 mg/m^3). Even for Germany, which sets the tightest OEL for nuisance dust, the OEL for respirable dust of 0.5 mg/m^3 (= 500 $\mu g/m^3$) is a factor of 10 higher than most of the daily limits for ambient $PM_{2.5}$ listed in Table 12.1. For the Unites States, the difference is even more than 100-fold. The rationale for this large difference is that even the most vulnerable parts of

Table 12.2: Legally binding occupational exposure limits (OELs) established in different countries for different types of dust.

Country/ agency	Material	Dust exposure limit (OEL) (mg/m³)		Comment
		Respirable[a]	Total[a]	
United States/ OSHA[b]	Nuisance dust	5	15	Dust without specific toxicity
	Carbon black		3.5	
	Cobalt, copper, vanadium		0.1–1.0	
	Quartz (silica)	0.05		
	Asbestos fibers	0.1 fib./cm³		
United States/ NIOSH[c]	TiO_2 (fine)	2.4		Not legally binding
	TiO_2 (ultrafine)	0.3		
EU	—	—	—	For some materials: upper limit of OEL for all EU countries are provided
	Crystalline TiO_2	0.1		
	Asbestos fibers	0.1 fib./cm³		
Germany	Nuisance dust	0.5	4	Respirable limits for particle density of 2.5 g/cm³
	Crystalline TiO_2	0.05		
	Quartz (silica)	0.05		
	Asbestos	0.1 fib./cm³		
Japan/ OSHA	Nuisance dust	2	8	Limestone, inorganic and organic dusts other than classes 1 and 2

(*Continued*)

Table 12.2: (*Continued*)

Country/ agency	Material	Dust exposure limit (OEL) (mg/m³)		Comment
		Respirable[a]	Total[a]	
	Class 2	1	4	Dusts containing less than 3% crystalline silica, bakelite, carbon black, coal, cork dust, cotton dust, iron oxide, grain dust, joss stick material dust, marble, portland cement, titanium oxide, zinc oxide
	Class 1	0.5	2	Activated charcoal, alumina, aluminum, bentonite, diatomite, graphite, kaolinite, pagodite, pyrites, pyrite cinder, talc
	Ferrovanadium	1		
	Quartz (silica)	0.03		
	Asbestos	0.003–0.15 fib./cm³		

[a]*Respirable* and *total* PM correspond approximately to $PM_{2.5}$ and PM_{10}, respectively, but the exact cut-off diameters vary, depending on the country.
[b]OSHA stands for Occupational Safety and Health Administration.
[c]NIOSH stands for National Institute for Occupational Safety and Health.

the population are exposed to ambient PM, while mostly young and healthy workers are hired to work under highly polluted workplace conditions. Moreover, in contrast to ambient PM, PM exposure at the workplace is limited to 8 h per day.

Another potentially harmful dust are fiber-like particles such as single-/double-walled carbon nanotubes (SWCNTs/DWCNTs), metal oxide fibers or all fibers meeting the so-called WHO criteria, i.e., fibers that are biopersistent (not efficiently dissolved or degraded within the biological matrix), rigid (not elastic), at least 5 µm long and fiber-like (i.e., length-to-diameter ratio is larger than 3). Especially for CNTs, there are numerous potential industrial applications including composite carbon materials (e.g., cars or aircrafts) and extremely stable concrete. Consequently, there have been numerous efforts of deriving suggestions for OEL, but only the British Standards Institute has put a legally binding OEL of 0.01 fiber/cm^3 into effect for the United Kingdom (Table 12.3). The other proposed OELs are mass-based and range from 1 to 50 µg/m^3 for entangled, non-rigid multi-walled CNTs manufactured by Bayer Inc. (Germany), the so-called Baytubes.

12.3 Shifting from Mass- to Surface Area-Derived OELs

For historic reasons and due to the well-established methods for accurate measurement of aerosol mass concentrations, all of the OELs presented above are based on PM mass concentration except for OELs for fibers, which are based on number concentration. Number-based dose metrics are justified for fiber-like particles (especially WHO fibers), as the proposed mode of action involves frustrated phagocytosis, which can potentially be induced by a single fiber independent of its mass or surface area (Chapter 10). On the other hand, for non-fiber particles, there is significant toxicological evidence that surface area (not mass) is the most relevant dose metric for PM-induced adverse health effects. In light of the emergence of a multitude of extremely diverse nanomaterials with a wide range of mass-specific surface areas (ca. 1–2000 m^2/g), various proposals for shifting from a mass- to a number or surface area-based hazard classification scheme have been put forward.[12]

This discussion has not yet resulted in a commonly accepted risk assessment scheme, but the conceptual approaches are converging toward the following numerical mass-to-surface area conversion scheme

Table 12.3: Suggested and (one) established occupational exposure limits for exposure to single- and multiwalled carbon nanotubes (SWCNT/MWCNT) and other fibers.

Material	Exposure limit ($\mu g/m^3$)	Comment	Reference
MWCNT ("Baytubes,"[a] highly agglomerated)	50	Suggested by industry (Bayer) based on 13-week rat inhalation study	4,5
	2	Scientific review of toxicological data (mainly rat inhalation studies)	6
MWCNT (BASF Nanocyl NC 7000)	2.5	Suggested by industry (BASF, Germany) based on 13-week rat inhalation study	7,8
	1	Scientific review of available toxicological data (mainly rat studies)	6
SWCNT and MWCNT	30	Based on a study funded by the Japanese Research Institute of Science for Safety and Sustainability, National Institute of Advanced Industrial Science and Technology Japan; based on 4-week rat inhalation study	3,9
CNT (SWCNT and MWCNT)	1	Exposure limit recommended (not legally binding) by the US National Institute for Occupational Safety and Health (NIOSH) based on available toxicological data from animal inhalation studies	10
SWCNT, MWCNT, metal oxide fibers, all WHO fibers[b]	0.01 fiber/cm³	Legally binding benchmark exposure limit established by the British Standards Institute (BSI); based on lung clearance rates of asbestos fibers	11

[a] *Baytubes* are MWCNTs developed and manufactured by Bayer Inc. (Germany), not produced anymore.
[b] WHO fibers: all fibers, which are biopersistent, rigid, >5 μm long, of diameter <3 μm and have length-diameter ratio >3.

$$\mathrm{OEL}_{SA,\,nd} = 10\,\frac{m^2}{g}\,\mathrm{OEL}_{M,nd}, \qquad (12.1a)$$

$$\mathrm{OEL}_{SA,x} = \mathrm{OEL}_{SA,nd}/f_{\mathrm{hazard},x}, \qquad (12.1b)$$

$$\mathrm{OEL}_{M,x} = \mathrm{OEL}_{SA,x}/\mathrm{BET}_x, \qquad (12.1c)$$

where Eq. (12.1a) adopts the already existing mass-based OEL for nuisance dust ($\mathrm{OEL}_{M,nd}$; see Table 12.2) and converts it into an equivalent surface area-based OEL ($\mathrm{OEL}_{SA,nd}$). Table 12.4 explains the choice of f_{hazard} and Brunauer-Emmett-Teller (BET) for different types of materials and toxicity classes (indicated by subscript x). In Eq. (12.1), one assumes that micron-sized nuisance dust has a mass-specific surface area of ca. 10 m²/g, which corresponds to particles with ca. 0.2 µm diameter (the size of maximum surface area concentration for urban aerosol; see Figure 9.1), having a material density of 3 g/cm³. For particles with diameters smaller than 0.2 µm (e.g., nanoparticles), smaller particle density and/or higher porosity, the mass-specific surface area, BET, will exceed 10 m²/g, which is accounted for by Eq. (12.1c) (see below). Eq. (12.1b) accounts for any material-specific toxicity as described the (surface area-based) hazard factor ($f_{\mathrm{hazard},x}$) given in Table 12.4. For BET, there is a standard measurement method utilizing the adsorption of inert gas molecules (e.g., argon or nitrogen) to powder particles.[13] For the determination of f_{hazard}, there is currently no standard method available. For demonstration of the usefulness of already existing f_{hazard}, the hazard factors derived from acute pulmonary inflammation as reported by Schmid and Stoeger (2016)[14] are utilized here (see Chapter 10; Figure 10.8).

For $f_{\mathrm{hazard},x} > 1$, the expected adverse health effects are more severe than those from nuisance dust. Similarly, for $f_{\mathrm{hazard},x} < 1$, less severe health effects are expected. Inhaled highly soluble particles (toxicity class I) are typically considered nontoxic ($f_{\mathrm{hazard},x} = 0$), because the material is quickly dissolved in body fluids and hence diluted to levels that are not expected to induce adverse health effects. For toxicity class IIa, micron-sized nuisance dust, $f_{\mathrm{hazard},x}$ is per definition equal to 1. However, there are materials with elevated material-specific toxicity (class III) such as some transition metals (IIIa) and crystalline quartz (IIIb). Of course, the list of class III materials is not complete; further class III materials (with material-specific toxicity) can be added by

Table 12.4: Calculation of OEL for nano-sized dust with and without material-specific toxicity, utilizing material-specific surface area and hazard factors (characteristic parameters required for Eq. (12.1)).

Class	Description	Mass-specific surface area (BET; m²/g)	Hazard factor (f_{hazard})	SA-derived respirable OEL (mg/m³)	Examples
I	Highly soluble materials (>dissolution limit in water > 100 mg/L = 100 µg/mL)	10[a]	0	0	Salt
IIa	Micron-sized nuisance dust with BET < 10 m²/g (corresponds to particle diameter ca. 0.2 µm; density ca. 3 g/cm³)	10[b]	1	5[c]	Low-solubility, low-toxicity materials including ambient PM (not ultrafine), polystyrene, amorphous SiO_2, TiO_2, Fe_xO_y (Chapter 10)
IIb	(Nano-sized) nuisance dust with high mass-specific surface area (BET > 10 m²/g; here: 10–100 m²/g)	Measured[b]	1	0.5–5	As class IIa but including nano-sized structures
IIIa	Materials with specific toxicity (e.g., release of metal ions, some transition metals)	Measured[b]	12[d]	0.04–0.4	Transition metals such as Zn-, Co- Cu-, Ni-oxides
IIIb	Crystalline quartz (lysosomal destabilization)	10[b]	60[d]	0.08[c]	Not a nanostructured material, i.e., per definition f_{SA} = 30 m²/g
IIIc	Materials with other material-specific toxicity pathways	Measured[b]	Measured[d]	—	
IV	WHO fibers	Number-based OEL 0.01 fiber/cm³			Biopersistent, rigid, length: >5 µm, diameter: <3 µm, length:diameter: >3:1

[a]For highly soluble materials, the mass-specific surface area is irrelevant (here, 10 was selected), as f_{hazard} = 0 implies that OEL is infinitely large (i.e., no health risk). OEL levels only apply to biopersistent materials (not highly soluble materials).

[b]The mass-specific BET surface area can be determined by a standard gas adsorption method, typically referred to as Brunauer–Emmett–Teller (BET) method.[13] For BET < 10 m²/g, BET = 10 m²/g is used; for BET > 10 m²/g, the measured value is used (10–100 m²/g is a realistic BET range for occupational settings).

[c]For class II and III materials, the OEL for nuisance dust is taken as starting point (here, the US value for respirable nuisance dust is taken; Table 12.2). Of course, the method can also be applied for a different "nuisance dust OEL" as established by different countries.

[d]The (surface area-based) hazard factors (f_{hazard}) are determined based on standardized (animal) experiments. There is no standard method available for this yet. For demonstration, values from acute inflammogenicity experiments in rodents are reported.[14]

[e]For crystalline quartz, which is not a nanostructured material (10 m²/g), the class IIa OEL is divided by f_{hazard} = 60.

experimentally determining their mass-specific surface area (BET) and hazard factor (f_{hazard}). Finally, class IV refers to WHO fibers. Their OEL is given not in terms of mass-based (or surface area-based) OEL, but in terms of number-based OEL for reasons described above.

We note that it is likely that there is a large overlap between "nuisance dust" materials and low-solubility, low toxicity (nano-)materials, although the former definition relates to regulatory measures on occupational PM and the latter was derived from toxicological studies with numerous materials (see Chapter 10).

As an application of this approach, we have calculated the surface area-derived OEL (see Table 12.4). For this, we assumed that the respirable OEL of the Unite States is valid (OEL_{IIa} = 5 mg/m^3) and then derived corresponding OEL values for different materials with known OEL, leveraging the surface-area based hazard factors from Figure 10.8. For nanostructured nuisance dust with an assumed (typical) mass-specific surface area of 10–100 m^2/g, Eq. 12 yields OEL_{IIb} = 0.5–5 mg/m^3. For material with additional toxicity such as transition metals (f_{hazard} = 12), the corresponding OEL_{IIIa} is 0.04–0.4 mg/m^3. For crystalline quartz, which typically has BET < 10 m^2/g, application of Eq. 12 implies that OEL_{IIa} has to be divided by f_{hazard} = 60, yielding OEL_{IIIb} = 0.08 mg/m^3.

The comparison of the OEL values derived from surface area-based toxicity considerations (Eq. 12 and Table 12.4) agree reasonably well with OEL values established in the United States for dust types other than nuisance dust (Table 12.2). The calculated OEL_{IIb} range of 0.5–5 mg/m^3 includes the (legally not binding) NIOSH limit value for fine TiO_2 and is ca. 5-fold less stringent than the corresponding NIOSH limit for "ultrafine TiO_2" (0.3 mg/m^3). For transition metal oxide, the surface area-derived OEL was determined as 0.04–0.4 mg/m^3 for respirable dust, which corresponds to 0.12–1.2 mg/m^3 for total dust. The latter is in excellent agreement with the US OEL of 0.1–1 mg/m^3. Similarly, the surface area-derived OEL for (respirable) quartz of 0.08 mg/m^3 is within expected experimental uncertainties, consistent with the US OEL of 0.05 mg/m^3.

Consequently, surface area-derived OEL holds the potential to provide reliable OEL for any arbitrary occupational setting purely based on the experimental determination of the mass-specific surface area and hazard factor. In light of the large diversity of nanomaterials, which are implemented in consumer products, this approach may be an important step toward "factory-specific" OEL with only requiring the measurement of BET and f_{hazard} for samples from each of the factories.

12.4 Successful PM Mitigation Strategies

The past decades have seen a significant reduction in ambient PM levels especially in but not limited to high-income countries. This progress is due to a concerted effort from many parts of the society. On its website, the WHO has pointed out numerous examples of successful mitigation of aerosol emission due to measures taken by the industry as well as in transport, urban planning, power generation and waste management (http://www.who.int/mediacentre/factsheets/fs313/en/, accessed 2 September 2014):

- **Indoor (private/industry)**
  - Use of hood or at least chimneys at the cooking place
  - Leave the room for cigarette smoking or vaping of e-cigarettes
  - Filtration of indoor air using electrostatic filters of room air or more efficient filter-equipped ventilation systems
  - Opening of the windows, if no other effective means of ventilation is available.
- **Industry**
  - Use of clean technologies that reduce industrial smokestack emissions.
  - Improved management of urban and agricultural waste, including capture of methane gas emitted from waste sites as an alternative to incineration (for use as biogas).
- **Transport**
  - Shifting to clean modes of power generation.
  - Prioritizing rapid urban transit, walking and cycling networks in cities as well as rail interurban freight and passenger travel.
  - Shifting to cleaner heavy-duty diesel vehicles and low-emission vehicles and fuels, including fuels with reduced sulfur content.

- **Urban planning**
  - Improving the energy efficiency of buildings (e.g., better insulation, solar panels).
  - Making cities more compact, and thus energy efficient.
- **Power generation**
  - Increased use of low-emission fuels and renewable combustion-free power sources (such as solar, wind or hydropower).
  - Co-generation of heat and power.
  - Distributed energy generation (e.g., mini-grids and rooftop solar power generation).
- **Municipal and agricultural waste management**
  - Improved strategies for waste reduction, waste separation, recycling and reuse or waste reprocessing.
  - Improved methods of biological waste management such as anaerobic waste digestion to produce biogas are feasible.
  - Low-cost alternatives to the open incineration of solid waste.
  - Where incineration is unavoidable, combustion technologies with strict emission controls are critical.

This list represents only a small selection of effective measures against PM air pollution. Additional essential ingredients for success are awareness of the problem, willingness to reduce air pollution, change habits and invest available funds into implementation of PM mitigation strategies.

References

1. Lin YL, Zou JL, Yang W, and Li CQ. (2018). A Review of recent advances in research on PM$_{2.5}$ in China. *Int. J. Environ. Res. Public Health* **15**: E438.
2. WHO. (2014). Indoor air quality guidelines: household fuel combustion. http://www.who.int/indoorair/guidelines/hhfc/en/, Accessed 25 July 2019.
3. Nakanishi J. (2011). Risk assessment of manufactured nanomaterials: Carbon nanotubes. Research Institute of Science for Safety and Sustainability, National Institue of Advanced Industrial Science and Technology, Japan.
4. Pauluhn J. (2010). Subchronic 13-week inhalation exposure of rats to multiwalled carbon nanotubes: toxic effects are determined by density of agglomerate structures, not fibrillar structures. *Toxicol. Sci.* **113**: 226–242.

5. Pauluhn J. (2010). Multi-walled carbon nanotubes (Baytubes (R)): Approach for derivation of occupational exposure limit. *Regul. Toxicol. Pharmacol.* **57**: 78–89.
6. Aschberger K, Johnston HJ, Stone V, Aitken RJ, Hankin SM, Peters SA, Tran CL, and Christensen FM. (2010). Review of carbon nanotubes toxicity and exposure–appraisal of human health risk assessment based on open literature. *Crit. Rev. Toxicol.* **40**: 759–790.
7. Ma-Hock L, Treumann S, Strauss V, Brill S, Luizi F, Mertler M, Wiench K, Gamer AO, van Ravenzwaay B, and Landsiedel R. (2009). Inhalation toxicity of multiwall carbon nanotubes in rats exposed for 3 months. *Toxicol. Sci.* **112**: 468–481.
8. Nanocyl. (2009). Responsible care and nanomaterials case study Nanocyl. Presentation at European Responsible Care Conference, Prague. Brussels, Belgium: The European Chemical Industry Council (CEFIC). Downloaded 11 November 2013: http://www.cefic.org/Documents/ResponsibleCare/04_Nanocyl.pdf.
9. Nakanishi J. (2011). Risk assessment of manufactured nanomaterials: "Approaches" — Overview of approaches and results. Research Institute of Science for Safety and Sustainability, National Institue of Advanced Industrial Science and Technology, Japan.
10. NIOSH. (2013). Occupational exposure to carbon nanotubes and nanofibers. U.S. National Institute of Occupational Safety and Health (NIOSH), Current Intelligence Bulletin **65**: 1–158.
11. BSI. (2007). Nanotechnologies — Part 2: Guide to safe handling and disposal of manufactured nanomaterials. British Standards Institute (BSI). PD 6699-2:2008. London, UK: BSI Group.
12. van Broekhuizen P, van Veelen W, Streekstra WH, Schulte P, and Reijnders L. (2012). Exposure limits for nanoparticles: Report of an international workshop on nano reference values. *Ann. Occup. Hyg.* **56**: 515–524.
13. Brunauer S, Emmet PH, and Teller E. (1938). Adsorption of gases in multimolecular layers. *J. Am. Chem. Soc.* **60**: 309–319.
14. Schmid O, and Stoeger T. (2016). Surface area is the biologically most effective dose metric for acute nanoparticle toxicity in the lung. *J. Aerosol. Sci.* **99**: 133–143.

Index

absorption, 93
accumulation mode, 134
acinus, 14
adverse outcome pathway (AOP), 173
aerodynamic diameter, 21, 37, 127, 134
aerosol bolus dispersion, 57, 101, 104
aerosol deposition, 26, 28, 49, 69, 87, 178
Aerosol-Derived Airway Morphometry (ADAM), 105
aerosol emission, 142, 204
aerosol exposure, 94, 137, 148, 151, 165
aerosol sources, 43, 134, 141, 145, 151
aerosol transport, 25, 73
agglomeration, 139, 188
airspace dimension assessment (AiDA), 105, 108
airway surface layer, 88, 89
albuterol, 114
alveolar clearance, 87, 96
alveolar deposition, 79, 156, 182

alveolar macrophages, 17, 87, 91, 152
alveolar-capillary membrane, 14
ambient aerosol, 133, 141, 145, 193
aperture plate, 121
Apollo, 187

β2 agonist, 113
bioaerosol, 139, 147
blood–gas barrier, 7, 14
bolus deposition, 53, 56, 180
bronchodilators, 113
Brownian diffusion, 28, 30, 70, 73, 77, 101, 105

carbon nanotube (CNT), 199
cascade impactors, 37, 47
cause of death, 164
central-to-peripheral ratio, 63, 64, 97, 183
chemical composition, 133, 138, 141, 151, 169, 194
chlorofluorocarbon (CFC), 123
cigarette smoking, 146, 153, 159, 164, 204

cilia, 16, 88
clearance kinetics, 96
clinical studies, 65, 117, 157, 165
coagulation, 74, 77, 138
coarse mode, 134, 139, 141, 145
coarse particles, 137, 148, 183
coincidence counting, 43, 65
collimator, 61
combustion particles, 139
computational fluid dynamics (CFD), 75
computational models, 69
conducting zone, 10
convective inhomogeneity, 104
convective mixing, 57, 70, 74, 101
cutoff diameter, 39

dead space, 12
diagnostic tool, 101
dichotomy, 9
diffusion, 7, 57, 140
diluter, 43
direct numerical simulation (DNS), 76
disability-adjusted life years (DALY), 162, 166
discrete models, 69
dispersion, 57, 75, 103
dose, 62, 119, 126, 137, 152, 157, 158, 160, 168, 193, 199
drag force, 28, 77
dry aerosol deposition, 141
dry powder inhalers, 118, 126

e-cigarette, 147, 204
effective airway diameter (EAD), 105
electrostatic precipitation, 31
elemental carbon, 139, 142

emission, 137, 144, 196, 204
enhanced diffusion, 179
epidemiology, 157, 160
Eulerian approach, 77
exposure limit, 70, 171, 194, 195
extrathoracic airway, 8, 71
extrathoracic upper airway, 78
extra-vehicular activity (EVA), 185

fibers, 31, 172, 196, 199, 202
fine, 119, 136, 141, 162, 182, 189, 193, 197, 203
fluorescent imaging, 68
fluorescent marker, 60
Fraunhofer scattering, 45
free-fall, 178

gadolinium (Gd), 67
gamma camera, 60, 95
gamma scintigraphy, 60, 95, 182
gas exchange, 7, 13, 16, 167
gas-to-particle conversion, 138, 143
gel layer, 16, 88
geometric diameter, 21, 23
geometric standard deviation (GSD), 24, 134
gravitational force, 28
gravitational sedimentation, 30, 56, 70, 108, 177, 182
great fog of London, 4

Hatch–Choate equations, 135, 157
health effects, 144, 151, 194, 196, 199
histogram, 63
hybrid models, 79
hydrofluoroalkane (HFA), 123
hypergravity, 104, 183

ICRP lung model, 70, 155
imaging, 59, 78, 95, 183
impaction, 39, 47, 126, 140
indoor aerosol, 133, 145
inertial impaction, 26, 28, 30, 32, 69, 105
inhaled antibiotics, 116
inhaled corticosteroids (ICS), 114
inhaled dose, 119
insulin, 117, 129
interception, 31
International Space Station, 185
intra-acinar, 78
intrinsic mobility, 101
intrinsic properties of the particles, 28, 101

key events, 173

LABA, 114
Lagrangian, 77
LAMA, 114
laminar flow, 26, 27, 76
large eddy simulation (LES), 76
laser-phase Doppler anemometry, 47
lognormal distribution, 21, 24, 134
Lorenz–Mie model, 46
low-angle light scattering, 45
lower respiratory tract (LRT), 70
lowered gas density, 186
lunar dust, 187
lymph nodes, 91
lymphatics, 87, 92

99mTc, 60, 64, 66, 95, 181, 182

Martian dust, 189
mass distribution, 22–25, 134, 135

mass median aerodynamic diameter (MMAD), 23, 134
microgravity, 104, 178, 182
MION, 68
mode shift, 55, 58
molecular initiating event (MIE), 173
monodisperse, 21, 25, 45, 49, 74, 105, 178
MPPD, 72
MRI, 66
mucociliary clearance (MCC), 17, 87, 88, 90, 152, 181
mucus glands, 16
mucus, 16, 88, 89, 95, 116, 155
multi-dimensional models, 75
multiple path particle deposition, 72

nasal olfactory mucosa, 94
Navier–Stokes equation, 76
near-Earth object (NEO), 190
nebulizers, 118, 120, 121, 128
next generation impactor (NGI), 37, 40
nicotine, 117
nitric oxide (NO), 115, 137, 167
nominal dose, 119
non-reversibility, 102, 180
nucleation mode, 133, 137
number distribution, 22, 24

occupational exposure limit (OEL), 194, 196, 197, 200
One-Dimensional Continuous Models, 73
organic, 137, 139, 142

parabolic flight, 178, 186
particle dissolution, 87

particle translocation, 93
particulate matter (PM), 4, 87, 95, 133, 144, 151, 163, 193
penetration volume (V_p), 54, 56, 75, 102, 180, 186
permissible exposure level (PEL), 188
phagocytosis, 17, 87, 91, 172
photochemical processing, 141, 144, 151
photomultiplier tube (PMT), 61
planar gamma scintigraphy, 60, 64
plume, 47, 123, 125
PM0.1, 4, 136, 137, 193
PM10, 4, 136, 137, 142, 146, 193
PM2.5, 4, 136, 137, 140, 142, 145, 162, 164, 193, 194, 198
pneumatic nebulizers, 118
polydisperse, 21, 25
positron emission tomography (PET), 65
premature deaths, 151, 162, 164
pressurized metered dose inhaler (pMDI), 3, 123
projection image, 62
prostacyclin analogs, 115
pulmonary arteries, 10, 13
pulmonary capillary, 14, 15
pulmonary interstitium, 92
pulmonary vasodilators, 113, 115
pulmonary veins, 10, 13

radioactive tracer, 60, 65
rain-out, 138, 139
regulatory, 4, 136, 169, 173, 174, 193, 194
resolution, 44, 62, 65, 69, 78, 106

respirable dose, 119
respiratory zone, 10, 13
resuspension, 139, 146
retention, 70, 87, 96, 97
Reynolds number, 26, 27
Reynolds-averaged Navier–Stokes (RANS), 76

salbutamol, 114
scattered light, 44, 50
scintillation, 61
second moment, 63
sedimentation, 2, 26, 28–30, 56, 58, 59, 70, 74, 77, 101, 108, 140, 177, 178, 182
settling velocity, 21, 30, 105
sheath flow, 41, 43
short-acting beta-agonist (SABA), 113, 114
short-acting muscarinic agent (SAMA), 114
single-photon emission computed tomography, 64
size distribution, 21, 22, 44, 134, 136, 140, 143, 155, 194
skew, 55, 63
smart nebulizers, 128
sol layer, 16, 18
soot, 138, 139, 144, 153, 165, 168, 170, 173
sources of urban aerosol, 140
spacer, 125
spacewalk, 185
spatial resolution, 62, 65–67, 69
SPECT, 64, 66
stochastic models, 73
Stokes number, 29, 39
structure of the lung, 7

superparamagnetic iron oxide particles, 68
surface area distribution, 22–24, 135, 136
systemic drug delivery, 117

Technicium-99, 60
third moment, 63
time-of-flight (TOF), 41, 42
total deposition, 32, 34, 49, 71, 74, 179, 182, 184
toxicity, 87, 169, 172, 187, 196, 201, 202
toxicology, 153, 157, 158, 168
trachea, 8, 16, 17, 27, 70, 88, 89, 181
tracheobronchial retention, 97
tubes, 198, 200
turbinates, 9
turbulence, 26, 31, 32, 76
turbulent flows, 31, 76
tyndallometer, 44, 47, 178

ultrafine particles, 94, 136
ultrasonic nebulizers, 120
upper airways, 8, 16, 127, 187
upper respiratory tract (URT), 30, 70
urban aerosol, 133, 136, 140, 156, 165, 201

vaccination, 117
valved holding chamber, 125
ventilation distribution, 66, 72, 101, 104
vibrating mesh nebulizers, 121

Whitby model, 134, 136

Years Lost due to Disabilities (YLD), 162
Years of Life Lost (YLL), 162

zero-g, 178, 184